Ethnic Dermatology

Ethnic Dermatology Clinical Problems and Skin Pigmentation

Second Edition

Clive B Archer

MD, PhD (Lond), FRCP Edin, FRCP (Lond)
Consultant Dermatologist and Honorary Clinical Senior Lecturer
Bristol Dermatology Centre
Bristol Royal Infirmary (UBHT) and
University of Bristol
Bristol
UK

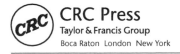

CRC Press
Taylor & Francis Group
Boca Raton London New York

CRC Press is an imprint of the
Taylor & Francis Group, an **informa** business

CRC Press
Taylor & Francis Group
6000 Broken Sound Parkway NW, Suite 300
Boca Raton, FL 33487-2742

First issued in paperback 2019

© 2008 by Taylor & Francis Group, LLC
CRC Press is an imprint of Taylor & Francis Group, an Informa business

The Author has asserted his right under the Copyright, Designs and Patents Act 1988 to be identified as the Author of this Work.

ISBN-13: 978-0-415-47119-0 (hbk)
ISBN-13: 978-0-367-38663-4 (pbk)

A CIP record for this book is available from the British Library.

Library of Congress Cataloging-in-Publication Data
Data available on application

**Visit the Taylor & Francis Web site at
http://www.taylorandfrancis.com**

**and the CRC Press Web site at
http://www.crcpress.com**

Contents

Preface   vii

1   Skin diseases and ethnic groups   1

2   Disorders with epidermal change   20

3   Disorders of the epidermal appendages and related disorders   52

4   Disorders of the dermal–epidermal interface and the dermis   67

5   Disorders of epidermal and dermal–epidermal cohesion: blistering disorders   77

6   Disorders of the dermis   87

7   Disorders of the vasculature and subcutaneous disorders   102

8   Dermatological aspects of internal medicine   110

9   Disorders of altered reactivity   126

10   Disorders of melanocytes   138

11   Non-melanocytic tumours   153

12   Infectious diseases and infestations   160

Index   193

Preface

Doctors outside dermatology are often surprised that there are nearly 2000 different skin diseases. Depending on variations in medical practice worldwide, skin disorders may present to a wide range of clinicians, including specialist dermatologists, trainee dermatologists, family practitioners (general practitioners), and hospital doctors, in addition to other healthcare workers.

The aims of this book on ethnic dermatology are to improve the diagnostic skills of doctors and other healthcare workers, not only in patients with 'white skin' (white Caucasians) but also in patients from different ethnic groups, and to provide an up-to-date approach to the investigation of patients with skin diseases, before making some therapeutic suggestions. I have used the term 'ethnic' to mean 'origin by birth or descent rather than nationality, relating to race or culture' and not to denote 'non-European'. The comparison of skin disorders in white and deeply pigmented skin is an important way of learning. By using this book regularly, the reader will become familiar with the appearance of common and uncommon skin diseases in people with varying degrees of skin pigmentation. Even 'white' skin is pigmented and different ethnic groups will have lighter or darker skin, ranging from the fair skin of Chinese Asians to the brown skin of Indian Asians to the dark brown, almost black skin of Afro-Caribbeans, African-Americans or Africans.

This book has evolved from *Black and White Skin Diseases: an Atlas and Text**. As in that book, I have defined deeply pigmented or 'black' skin broadly to include people of African, Black or African-American, Afro-Caribbean, Indian or Australasian origin.

From an early stage in my dermatology training, I realized that those dermatologists who were best at diagnosing skin diseases in deeply pigmented skin were those with most experience of such patients, a fact which is hardly surprising. This observation was reinforced when I later spent some time in Ethiopia, where I met a number of European doctors working in various parts of Africa. 'We know very well how to recognize leprosy' one of them said, 'but when it comes to even the commonest of other skin diseases, we have great difficulty, since nearly all of our medical school dermatology teaching was in white skin'.

Recognizing the enormous variety of skin diseases in white skin depends on the development of a number of visual skills that have to be developed still further to recognize skin diseases in deeply pigmented skin from different ethnic groups. The purpose of this book is to present a systematic approach to the diagnosis of a wide range of skin diseases seen in black and white skin. It is not intended to be a comprehensive atlas of tropical medicine, but one should always consider the possibility of diseases such as leprosy in patients who have lived in tropical countries.

I began *Black and White Skin Diseases* when working at the St John's Institute of Dermatology in London. I was appointed as Consultant Dermatologist and Honorary Clinical Senior Lecturer at Bristol Royal Infirmary (UBHT) and the University of Bristol in 1989. I am most grateful to the medical photographer **Stuart Robertson** of the Department of Education at the St John's Institute of Dermatology, St Thomas' Hospital, London for his invaluable help, and to the Consultant staff of St John's, past and present, for access to the collection of photographs at the St John's Institute of Dermatology.

In my time as Academic Vice President of the British Association of Dermatologists, I would like to acknowledge those who most influenced my early dermatology

*Archer CB, Robertson SJ. Black and White Skin Diseases: an Atlas and Text. Oxford: Blackwell Science, 1995.

thinking, in particular Mac (DM) MacDonald, Charles (RS) Wells, and Rod Hay of Guy's Hospital, London, and Malcolm Greaves, Etain Cronin, Gerald Levene, Neil Smith, and Edward Wilson Jones of the St John's Institute of Dermatology, London. Many photographs are from the collection in Bristol and I am most grateful for the support of my colleagues in the Departments of Dermatology and Medical Illustration and Photography. Before moving to Bristol, I spent a most interesting 2 years as Research Fellow with Jon Hanifin at the Oregon Health Sciences University, Portland and was much influenced by the systematic approach to the teaching and learning of dermatology in the USA.

Clive B Archer
2008

CHAPTER 1

Skin diseases and ethnic groups

SKIN PIGMENTATION
DERMATOLOGICAL PROBLEMS IN BLACK SKIN
Diagnostic difficulties
Pigmentary responses to diseases or treatments
Prominent follicular and dermal inflammation
NORMAL VARIANTS IN BLACK SKIN
CLINICAL ASSESSMENT
Dermatological history
General history
  Past medical history

Family history
Social history
Examining the patient
  Morphology
  Distribution
Clinical investigations
  Dermatoscopy
  Wood's light
  The 'acarus hunt'

Dermatology is historically a general medical specialty, supported by a broad range of clinical and basic science research. In recent years there has been an increasing emphasis on the surgical aspects of managing skin disorders. This trend is partly due to the success of skin cancer public information programmes. Dermatology continues to be one of the most popular career options amongst young doctors worldwide.

The aim of this book on ethnic dermatology is to improve the diagnostic and investigation skills of doctors and other healthcare workers, not only in patients with 'white skin' (white Caucasians) but also in patients from different ethnic groups. I have used the term 'ethnic' to denote 'origin by birth or descent rather than nationality, relating to race or culture'. By using this book regularly, the reader will become familiar with the appearance of common and uncommon skin diseases in people with varying degrees of skin pigmentation. Even 'white' skin is pigmented, and different ethnic groups will have more deeply pigmented skin, ranging from the fair skin of Chinese Asians to the brown skin of Indian Asians to the dark brown, almost black skin of Afro-Caribbeans, African-Americans or Africans. I have defined deeply pigmented or 'black' skin broadly to include people of African, Black or African-American, Afro-Caribbean, Indian, or Australasian origin.

Recognizing the enormous variety of skin diseases in white skin depends on the development of a number of visual skills, which have to be developed still further to recognize skin diseases in deeply pigmented skin from different ethnic groups. Since the number of different skin diseases has been estimated at nearly 2000, one should not expect to develop instant expertise. For example, it is possible to manage a patient appropriately without detailed knowledge of all of the benign adnexal tumours, but I am afraid the old adage that 'there are only two skin diseases, those that are steroid-responsive and those that are not' does display a rather outdated lack of learning! A reasonable knowledge of dermatology is essential for all doctors who look after patients.

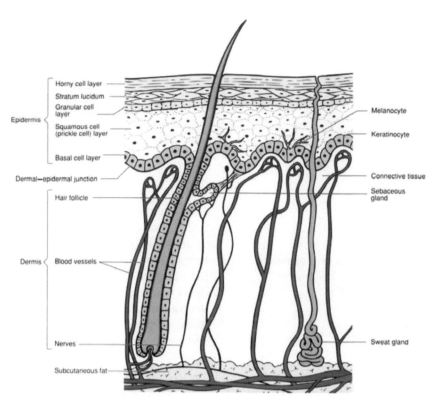

Figure 1.1   Diagramatic view of the skin.

Skin diseases are common, accounting for about 15% of family practitioner (general practitioner) consultations.

Commonly seen skin disorders include the inflammatory dermatoses (psoriasis, eczema/dermatitis, and urticaria), acne vulgaris, and benign and malignant skin tumours. Most rashes are recognized by the distribution of the eruption, the history being used for fine-tuning: e.g. in deciding on the distinction between endogenous and exogenous eczema. Redness or erythema can be helpful in identifying inflammatory diseases but this sign may be difficult to assess in deeply pigmented or black skin. If the diagnosis is not obvious, it can be useful to consider which level of the skin is involved in the pathological process (e.g. is this an epidermal or dermal problem?) (Figure 1.1). Table 1.1 shows a simplified classification of skin diseases according to the predominant level of pathology in the skin, although in some disorders more than one level will be involved. A list of commonly used dermatology terms is shown in Table 1.2.

SKIN PIGMENTATION

Although the density of melanocytes in the basal layer of the epidermis varies between different sites on the body, this value for a particular site of skin remains relatively constant in the different ethnic or racial groups. Melanin is produced at the site of the cytoplasmic melanosomes, which are subsequently transferred from the melanocyte to neighbouring keratinocytes. Differences in skin pigmentation depends on the size, shape, and distribution of the melanosomes, particularly their packaging within the keratinocytes. In white skin the melanosomes are

Table 1.1   Skin diseases according to the level of pathology in the skin

Predominant change/site of pathology	Disease
Epidermal changes (e.g. scaling, hyperkeratosis, crusting)	Psoriasis, eczema/dermatitis, superficial fungal infections, the ichthyoses
Epidermal appendages	Acne vulgaris, rosacea, hidradenitis suppurativa, alopecia areata
Dermal–epidermal interface and dermis	Pityriasis rosea, lichen planus, lupus erythematosus, erythema multiforme
Epidermal and dermal–epidermal cohesion (blistering disorders)	Pemphigus vulgaris/foliaceus, pemphigoid, dermatitis herpetiformis, epidermolysis bullosa
Dermis	The urticarias, granuloma annulare, scleroderma, dermatomyositis, lymphoma (e.g. cutaneous T-cell lymphoma), xanthoma/xanthelasma
Subcutaneous fat	Erythema nodosum and other forms of panniculitis

Table 1.2   Dermatological terminology

Lesion	Any single area of skin pathology
Macule	An area of colour change
Papule	An elevated (palpable) lesion less than 5 mm in diameter
Nodule	An elevated spherical lesion 5 mm or more in diameter, often extending deeply into the skin
Wheal (weal)	An oedematous slightly raised lesion, often with a pale centre and red margin
Plaque	A flat-topped palpable lesion usually more than 2 cm in diameter
Vesicle	A fluid-filled blister less than 5 mm in diameter
Pustule	A blister containing fluid with neutrophils (pus)
Bulla	A fluid-filled blister 5 mm or more in diameter
Purpura	A visible collection of free red blood cells in the skin
Scale	Thickened fragments of the outermost layer of the epidermis, the stratum corneum
Crust	Dried plasma exudate
Excoriation	An abrasion caused by scratching
Lichenification	An area of increased epidermal thickness and increased skin markings as a result of chronic rubbing
Erosion	An absence of the epithelial surface
Ulcer	An absence of the epithelial surface with dermal damage (i.e. deeper than an erosion)
Scar	A permanent lesion resulting from repair by replacement with connective tissue
Telangiectasia	Dilated blood vessels visible on the skin surface

small and tend to be in membrane-bound complexes of 3 or more, whereas in black skin the melanosomes are larger, elliptical, single bodies, which can be found intact in the stratum corneum. In other words, racial differences in pigmentation are due to differences in melanogenesis and not due to altered melanocyte numbers. The melanin in the skin is photo-protective. Table 1.3 shows a classification of

Table 1.3 Skin types according to sun reactivity and pigmentary response

Skin type	Sun reactivity	Pigmentary response
I	Very sensitive; always burns easily	Little or no tan
II	Very sensitive; always burns	Minimal tan
III	Sensitive; burns moderately	Tans gradually (light brown)
IV	Moderately sensitive; burns minimally	Tans easily (brown)
V	Minimally sensitive; rarely burns	Tans darkly (dark brown)
VI	Not sensitive; never burns	Deeply pigmented (black)

skin types according to sun reactivity and pigmentary response.

DERMATOLOGICAL PROBLEMS IN BLACK SKIN

Dermatological problems in patients with deeply pigmented skin include diagnostic difficulties, pigmentary responses to diseases or treatments, and a tendency to prominent follicular and dermal inflammation (e.g. scarring and granulomatous diseases).

Diagnostic difficulties

So many inflammatory skin diseases present with redness or erythema but, as mentioned earlier, this sign may be difficult to assess in black skin. The difficulties in deeply pigmented skin regarding erythema are shown in Figure 1.2a and b, both of which are examples of an annular erythema. In Figure 1.2b, no erythema can be seen and the diagnosis is made from the annular appearance of the eruption accompanied by fine scaling, typical of this reactive dermatosis, and the knowledge that in black patients one often sees marked post-inflammatory hyperpigmentation, as opposed to any redness.

However, even in deeply pigmented skin, close inspection can sometimes reveal erythema, as seen in Figure 1.3a, a case of pityriasis rosea, confirmed by the 'Christmas tree' distribution of the eruption on the trunk (Figure 1.3b).

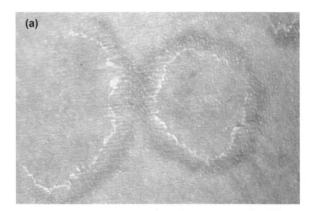

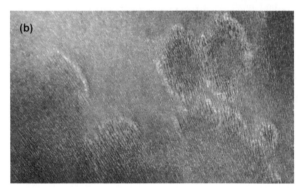

Figure 1.2a and b Annular erythema. (1.2a) A typical example in white skin. No erythema is seen in black skin (1.2b) but the lesions are annular, with fine scaling and post-inflammatory hyperpigmentation. Skin scrapings for mycology were negative.

To the experienced eye, many dermatological diagnoses are instantly recognizable but many doctors, with only limited medical school dermatology

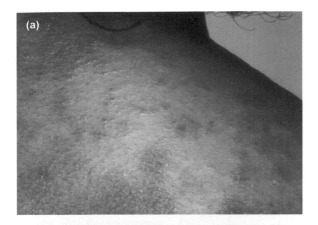

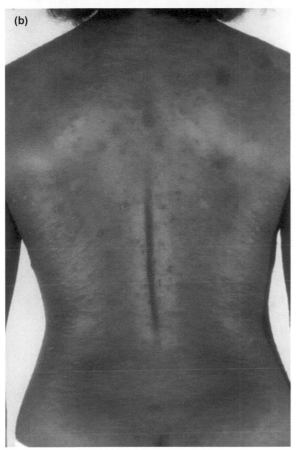

Figure 1.3a and b Pityriasis rosea. (1.3a) Close inspection of the hyperpigmented lesions in this West Indian woman revealed some erythema. (1.3b) The confirmatory 'Christmas tree' pattern of the eruption on the trunk.

teaching and learning to recall, will have little or no idea. All is not lost! Typical examples of granuloma annulare and annular sarcoidosis are shown in Figure 1.4a and b. In each of these cases there is no involvement of the outer layer of the skin (e.g. no scaling or other epidermal changes) and we are dealing with a dermal problem, the lesions being quite obviously circular in shape. One can then use a book such as this (or rely on one's memory or the internet) to compile a list of the differential diagnosis of annular dermal lesions. It requires a little more learning to know that granuloma annulare often occurs on the dorsa of the hands and that cutaneous sarcoidosis is commoner in black skin. In each case the diagnosis can be confirmed by a skin biopsy.

Pigmentary responses to diseases or treatments

Post-inflammatory hyperpigmentation (hypermelanosis) and post-inflammatory hypopigmentation (hypomelanosis) pose particular problems for black patients. In inflammatory disorders such as atopic dermatitis (Figure 1.5), acne vulgaris (Figure 1.6), and lichen planus (Figure 1.7), the post-inflammatory hyperpigmentation can persist well after the active disease process has subsided and sometimes indefinitely. Post-inflammatory hyperpigmentation particularly occurs in diseases that affect the basal layer of the epidermis, such as lichen planus (Figure 1.8) or lupus erythematosus (Figure 1.9), when melanin spills into the upper dermis to be engulfed by macrophages (pigmentary incontinence). Inflammatory skin diseases, such as psoriasis and atopic dermatitis, often lead to post-inflammatory hypopigmentation (Figure 1.10), thought to be due to the increased mitotic rate of keratinocytes and a decreased transit time of these cells to the skin surface before shedding. This results in diminished transfer of melanosomes from the melanocytes. Post-inflammatory hyper- and hypopigmentation are sometimes seen together (Figure 1.11). Black patients sometimes

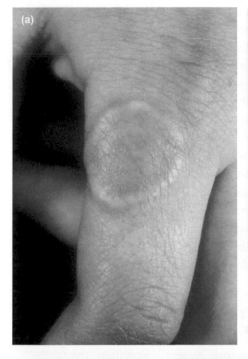

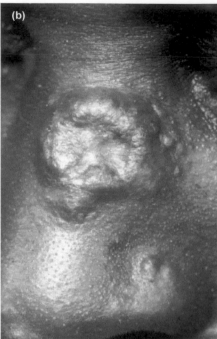

Figure 1.4a and b Granuloma annulare (1.4a) and annular sarcoidosis (1.4b) are predominantly dermal lesions. Granuloma annulare frequently occurs on the dorsa of the hands and cutaneous sarcoidosis is relatively common in black skin, particularly on the face.

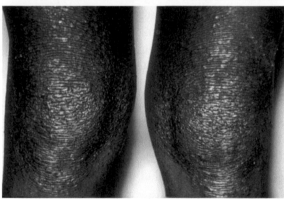

Figure 1.5 Atopic dermatitis, showing prominent lichenification (epidermal thickening and increased skin markings) and post-inflammatory hyperpigmentation on the knees.

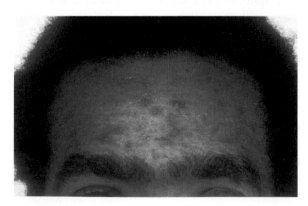

Figure 1.6 Acne vulgaris on the forehead. Post-inflammatory hyperpigmentation can last for months after active papules, pustules, nodules or cysts have ceased to develop, and sometimes persists indefinitely.

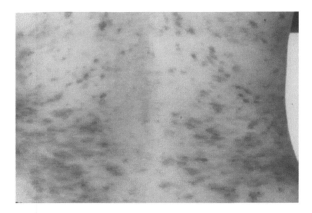

Figure 1.7 Lichen planus pigmentosus. Persistent marked hyperpigmentation on the lower back of an Indian man. The pigmentation may or may not be preceded by typical lichen planus.

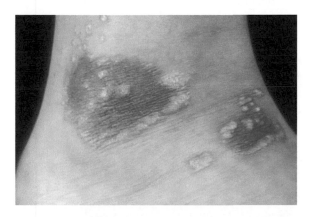

Figure 1.8 Annular lichen planus affecting the ankle region, showing some reddish-purple lesions, annular hyperkeratosis, and marked hyperpigmentation.

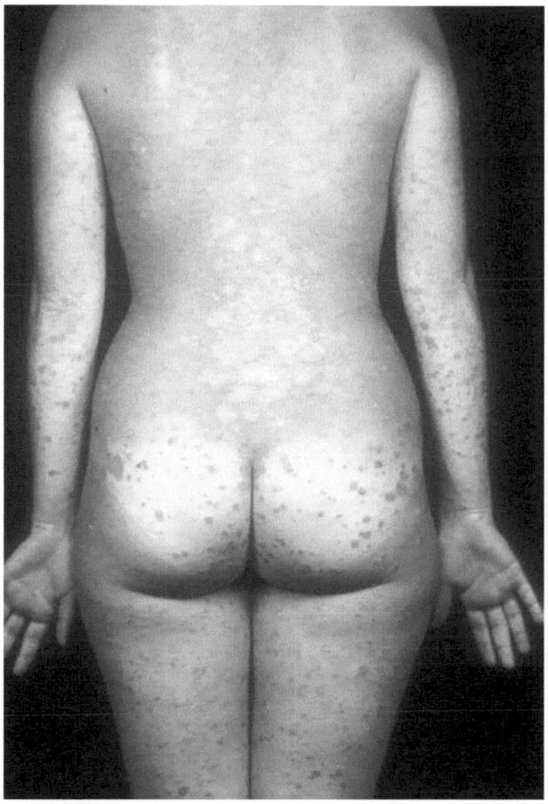

Figure 1.10 Psoriasis. This woman has inflammatory guttate lesions on the trunk, buttocks, and limbs, with post-inflammatory hypopigmentation on her previously sun-tanned back.

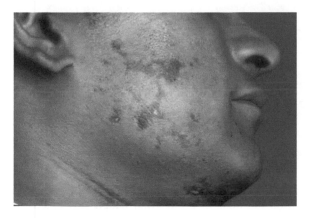

Figure 1.9 Chronic discoid lupus erythematosus, showing prominent post-inflammatory hyperpigmentation on the face in a man with deeply pigmented skin.

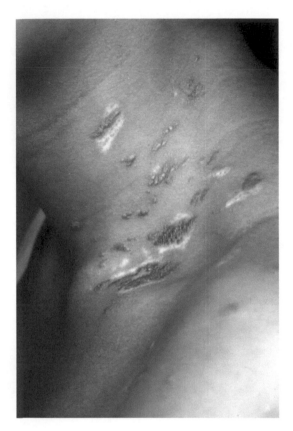

Figure 1.11 Lichen planus on the neck of a black patient, showing coexistent post-inflammatory hyperpigmentation and hypopigmentation.

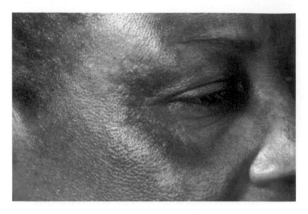

Figure 1.12 Acquired ochronosis on the cheek; the increased skin pigmentation results from the application of an over-the-counter skin lightening cream in a woman of West Indian origin. (Courtesy of Dr MJ Tidman.)

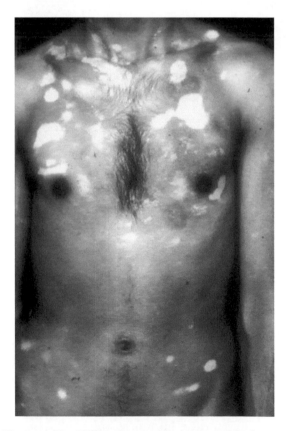

Figure 1.13 Vitiligo. Symmetrical areas of depigmentation on the trunk of a man with deeply pigmented skin.

use over-the-counter bleaching creams, containing hydroquinone, which can paradoxically lead to an increase in skin pigmentation, termed exogenous or acquired ochronosis (Figure 1.12).

Disorders of pigmentation are particularly noticeable in deeply pigmented skin. The depigmentation (as opposed to hypopigmentation) of vitiligo (Figure 1.13), in particular, can be very disfiguring, sometimes severely affecting the quality of people's lives. The superficial fungal infection, pityriasis versicolor (tinea versicolor) can induce decreased or increased skin pigmentation in black or white patients (Figure 1.14a and b).

In black patients papulosquamous diseases, such as psoriasis, frequently have a violaceous colour, with an overlying grey scale, and the distribution of the

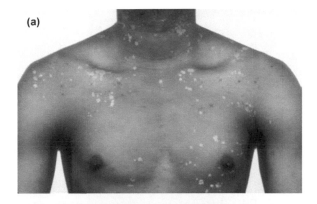

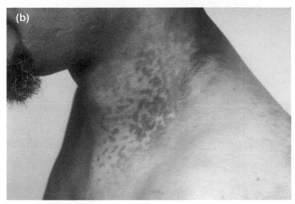

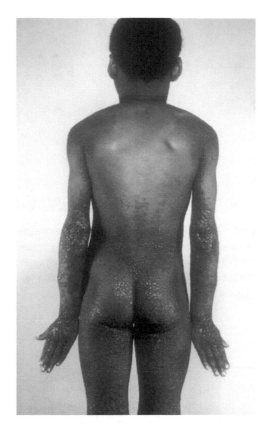

Figure 1.14a and b Pityriasis (tinea) versicolor, affecting the trunk and neck. Proliferation of yeasts may lead to hypopigmentation (1 14a) or hyperpigmentation (1.14b), particularly noticeable in black patients. Individual lesions coalesce to form confluent areas and close inspection may reveal fine scaling.

Figure 1.15 Atopic dermatitis, showing the 'reverse pattern' in a boy of West Indian origin, with thick lichenified lesions over the elbows and on the extensor surfaces.

eruption is an important factor in making a diagnosis. The distribution of the lesions may be different from the characteristic pattern in white skin, as seen with atopic dermatitis, in which the elbows, knees, and extensor aspects of the limbs can be involved in the so-called 'reverse pattern' (Figure 1.15).

Prominent follicular and dermal inflammation

Prominent follicular inflammation is regularly encountered in patients of African, Afro-Caribbean, or African-American origin. This can be seen in common diseases such as atopic dermatitis, in which the lesions can be accentuated around hair follicles (follicular

eczema) (Figure 1.16), or in uncommon diseases almost exclusive to black skin, such as disseminate and recurrent infundibulo-folliculitis (see Chapter 2). Figure 1.17a and b show examples of pseudofolliculitis barbae in which the shaved, curved hairs have penetrated the skin to set up a foreign body reaction, resulting in papules, pustules, and sometimes prominent post-inflammatory hyperpigmentation.

Examples of prominent dermal inflammation include keloidal scarring and sarcoidosis, which occur more frequently in black skin. Keloids, either induced by trauma (Figure 1.18a) or spontaneous (Figure 1.18b), can be devastating to the patient and very difficult to treat. Cutaneous sarcoidosis can be part of a systemic disease or can present with

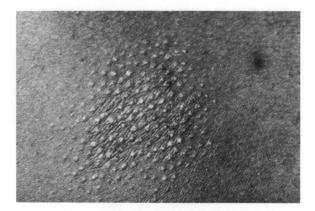

Figure 1.16 Follicular pattern of atopic dermatitis, showing grey scales overlying post-inflammatory hyperpigmentation. The eczematous lesions are accentuated around hair follicles. This pattern occurs more commonly in deeply pigmented skin.

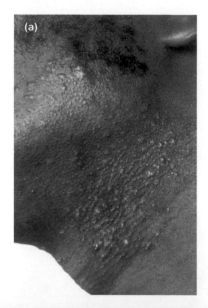

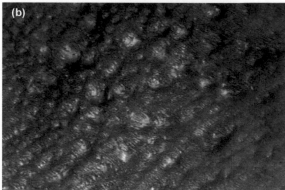

Figure 1.17a and b Pseudofolliculitis barbae, affecting the face and neck. This is relatively common in black men, in whom the shaved hairs penetrate the skin to set up a foreign body reaction, resulting in papules, pustules, and often prominent post-inflammatory hyperpigmentation.

skin involvement only (see Chapter 8). Discoid lupus erythematosus has no particular racial predilection, but causes prominent scarring and disfiguring post-inflammatory hyper- and/or hypopigmentation in black skin (see Chapter 8). One should always consider the possibility of diseases such as leprosy in patients who have lived in tropical countries.

NORMAL VARIANTS IN BLACK SKIN

Black patients sometimes present with skin problems that occur so commonly in black skin that they are considered to be normal variants. These include:

- palmar pits (keratosis punctata) in the skin creases, which themselves are sometimes darkly pigmented (Figure 1.19)
- asymptomatic pigmentation of the oral mucosa (Figure 1.20)
- nail pigmentation.

The latter may be seen as dark (occasionally black) linear longitudinal bands or streaks, diffuse dark pigmentation, or as exogenous pigmentation, as shown in Figure 1.21, following the use of henna. Darkly pigmented longitudinal lesions can also be caused by a benign melanocytic naevus (Figure 1.21), subungual malignant melanoma being uncommon in black skin. Other normal variants include hyperpigmented macules on the soles of the feet (Figure 1.22), Futcher's or Voigt's line of demarcation between dark and light skin on the upper arms (Figure 1.23) and midline hyperpigmentation or hypopigmentation over the sternum.

Cupping, a commonly practiced medical treatment in the Western hemisphere in the past, is still extensively used in developing countries and leads to characteristic hyperpigmented lesions (Figure 1.24).

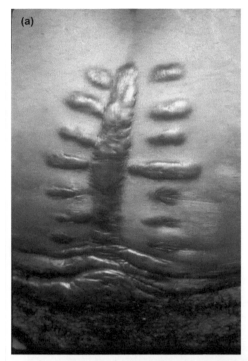

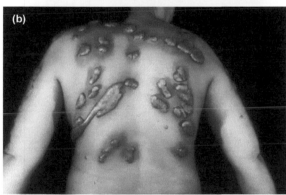

Figure 1.18a and b   Keloids. (1.18a) Marked keloid formation as a result of an abdominal operation. (1.18b) Keloids may also arise spontaneously (with no apparent preceding trauma or inflammation). Note the surrounding hyperpigmentation in this patient of North African origin.

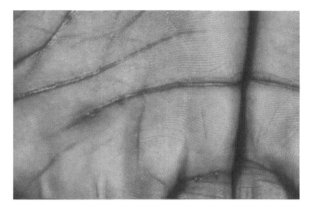

Figure 1.19   Palmar pits, occurring in the darkly pigmented skin creases of a man of West Indian origin. Palmar pits are commonly seen as a normal variant in black skin.

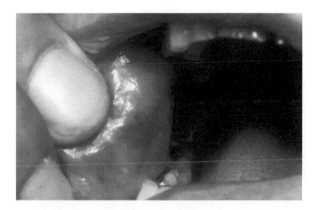

Figure 1.20   Pigmentation of the oral mucosa. Asymptomatic buccal pigmentation is common in people with black skin and does not necessarily represent post-inflammatory hyperpigmentation from a disease such as lichen planus.

One should always consider the possibility of diseases such as leprosy (Figure 1.25) or leishmaniasis in patients who have lived in tropical countries.

CLINICAL ASSESSMENT

As in other aspects of medicine, the diagnosis of skin disorders depends on taking a detailed but well-directed or focused history followed by examination of the patient and sometimes the performance of simple bedside tests and/or further clinical investigations. In order to maintain one's interest amidst busy clinics, it can be fun to guess the diagnosis from the referral letter, but this activity should never replace the sound clinical skills of history taking and clinical examination. There is usually no time for an exhaustive general medical history, and in many instances this would be inappropriate. However, one should avoid considering the dermatological problem in

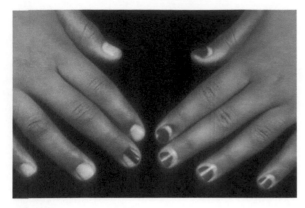

Figure 1.21 Nail pigmentation. This dark linear longitudinal band, in this case a melanocytic naevus, was seen on the right middle fingernail of a young West Indian woman, who also had exogenous pigmentation (henna) of the nails of the left hand.

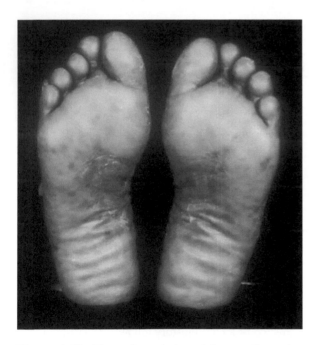

Figure 1.22 Hyperpigmented macules on the soles of the feet, incidentally occurring in a man of Afro-Caribbean origin with some scaling of the skin.

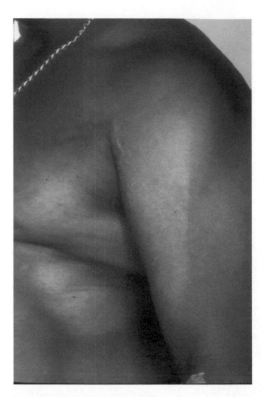

Figure 1.23 Futcher's or Voigt's line of demarcation between dark skin laterally and light skin medially on the upper arms is common in patients with deeply pigmented skin.

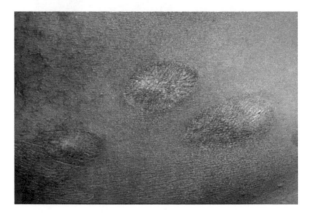

Figure 1.24 Cupping, showing characteristic hyperpigmented lesions on the trunk of an African man.

isolation from the patient's general medical setting and social circumstances. The consultation should allow sufficient time not only to make the correct diagnosis but also to explain to the patient, in terms that can be understood, the natural history and management of the particular skin disorder.

With experience, the referral letter or an early glimpse of the skin disorder can allow one to focus the history

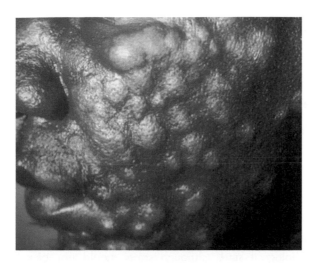

Figure 1.25 Lepromatous leprosy in a man of African origin. The occurrence of infiltrated lesions on the forehead provoked the clinical description of leonine facies (Chapter 12).

and, in some cases, the history will allow fine-tuning of the diagnosis. For example, a detailed personal, family, and social history will help the clinician decide whether a patient with hand eczema has exogenous or endogenous hand eczema, possibly a manifestation of atopic dermatitis (atopic eczema). An important function of taking a history is to allow the establishment of a rapport between the doctor and patient before the clinical examination is performed.

Dermatological history

Having established the age, sex, and racial origin of the patient and sometimes being led by the referral letter, I usually ask the patient to:

Describe in your own words what has been troubling you with your skin and when it started.

Patients vary in their ability to tell a concise, relevant story and the need for the doctor to tactfully interrupt will depend on this ability. It is usually possible to establish quickly whether one is dealing with a rash (such as eczema or psoriasis) or a skin lesion or lesions.

Dermatologists do not favour use of the term 'skin rash', and will offer cogent arguments based on the

fact that, to their knowledge, rashes do not affect other organs of the body. One should try to avoid asking leading questions but we all do it. Patients sometimes use words incorrectly. For example, a patient with urticaria may describe a wheal as a 'blister' and close questioning is required to establish that the patient has not actually seen any 'fluid-filled cavities'.

Helpful prompts include:

How did it start?
What did it look like?
How did it develop?
When exactly did it begin?
Have you had this before?
Did anything make it worse or better?

For example, did the rash begin in the summer and only occur on sunny days? Could the rash be related to the ingestion of a food or a recently prescribed drug? A list of concurrent medications and when each was started should help answer this question.

One should ask about previous treatments, especially topical treatments, either prescribed or purchased as over-the-counter preparations. Some of these treatments may have helped, whereas others may have made matters worse. For example, a potent fluorinated topical corticosteroid is sometimes erroneously applied to the face, leading to a perioral dermatitis; a fungal infection of the skin may worsen after the application of a topical corticosteroid, producing tinea incognita; or the patient may have become allergic to a local anaesthetic or preservative in a topical preparation used to alleviate pruritus ani.

It can be useful to ask early on:

Was the rash itchy?

and

Did the skin become dry, scaly, flaky, crusted or weepy?

Itching in the absence of epidermal changes is often due to urticaria and the history of intermittent whealing, of variable duration, sometimes associated with subcutaneous swelling (angioedema) may become evident. Severely itchy, excoriated, crusted skin may be due to a form of eczema or the mite infestation, scabies. Any suspicion of scabies should lead to the question:

Are any other family members or friends itching?

Generalized pruritus, in the absence of any rash or skin lesions, would lead one to consider general medical causes of itching.

If it becomes apparent that the presenting complaint is a skin lesion, either a benign or malignant skin tumour, the history is often directed by the clinical impression gained from an early glimpse of the lesion. The history of a slowly enlarging lesion developing over a few months on a sun-exposed site would be consistent with a basal cell carcinoma (BCC) or squamous cell carcinoma, whereas a rapidly growing lesion developing over a period of a few weeks would be more consistent with a keratoacanthoma. A rapid diagnosis of viral warts or molluscum contagiosum warts may render a detailed history unnecessary but, particularly in an adult, one might need to consider the possibility of immunosuppression and question the patient appropriately.

With increased awareness of the dangers of excessive sun exposure, patients are often concerned about the possibility of a benign melanocytic naevus or naevi changing into a malignant melanoma. Specific questions may include:

How long have you had this mole?
In what way has it changed?
Over what period of time?
Has it become larger?
Has it changed shape or color?
Has it bled or become itchy?

Spontaneous bleeding of a melanocytic lesion is more worrying than bleeding as a result of minor injury. In my experience, itching alone is usually not a sign of malignant change, but this symptom would take on more significance in the presence of other changes. Again, one should try to avoid leading the patient too much in a particular direction and, in this instance, the clinical appearance of the pigmented lesion or lesions will be particularly important. For example, these changing features would be perfectly acceptable in a seborrheic keratosis, which may be one of multiple lesions as one sees with benign melanocytic naevi.

General history

With experience, the general history will become well-directed as a result of information gained from the dermatological history. If necessary, one should ask further questions related to past medical history, family history, and social history, including occupation, leisure activities, home situation, and travel overseas. One should also form an opinion about the patient's psychological state, although stress should not be blamed too readily as the cause of the skin disease.

Past medical history

An exhaustive history of past medical illnesses is not always required, and this aspect of the consultation should be directed, to an extent, by the presenting complaint. A previous history of skin diseases such as psoriasis or eczema may be relevant or incidental to the present problem. If early impressions point to a form of eczema, perhaps atopic dermatitis, one should ask specifically about childhood eczema, asthma or hay fever. A patient with alopecia areata may also have vitiligo or other autoimmune diseases, including thyroiditis, diabetes mellitus, and pernicious anaemia.

Inquiry about past medical illnesses should include a history of prescribed drugs and over-the-counter medications. A general medical disease may be directly relevant to the dermatological disorder. For example, long-standing arthritis may prove to be psoriatic rather than another seronegative arthritis after all, and gastric symptoms may underlie iron deficiency anaemia with resultant diffuse hair loss.

Family history

Questions related to family history frequently follow on from the past medical history. There may well be a family history of psoriasis, atopic disorders or autoimmune diseases. It is important to take care in the interpretation of this aspect of the patient's history, however. The apparent occurrence of 'allergies' within the family can be particularly misleading.

A patient with an inherited disease such as neurofibromatosis may not volunteer a family history. Not all familial diseases are genetic in origin and a family history of pruritus in a patient with scabies may only become apparent on direct questioning.

Social history

The social history should include details of occupation, leisure activities, the home situation, and travel abroad.

When the occupation seems to be relevant to the skin disorder, as may be the case in hand eczema, one should find out precisely what the patient does at work. What materials are handled? Are protective clothing and/or gloves worn? What are the gloves made of? Sometimes a work-related skin disorder will settle down when the patient is absent from work, either on sick leave or on holiday. This is not always true, however, the chronic hand eczema of chromate sensitivity in cement workers being well known to persist after the allergen has been removed from the patient or vice versa.

Individuals with a background of atopic dermatitis or other manifestations of atopy, however mild, may develop severe, persistent hand eczema as hairdressers, caterers or nurses. This emphasizes the need for good career advice during the teenage years.

Leisure activities are an important aspect of most people's lives. Sporting activities may be associated with exacerbations of skin disorders. For example, sweating may irritate the skin of patients with atopic dermatitis, exercise can induce cholinergic urticaria, and impetigo can run riot in a rugby scrum! Hobbies such as photography can lead to the handling of irritant or sensitizing chemicals. One should enquire about personal habits, including the application of cosmetics (i.e. make-up, perfume, nail varnish, aftershave) the wearing of costume jewellery, and the colouring of hair.

A dusty home environment can cause exacerbations of atopic dermatitis, as can cigarette smoke. The home situation may be an important factor in the management of patients with skin disorders. Some patients will be unable to adequately treat their skin at home, either through lack of amenities, such as a bath, or because of a busy or disorganized lifestyle.

A knowledge of recent travel abroad, even for a short time, may be crucial to making the correct diagnosis. For example, it is not uncommon to see the occasional traveller with leishmaniasis or a tourist with cutaneous larva migrans (creeping eruption).

Examining the patient

Physical examination of the patient is an important part of making the correct diagnosis. One should always consider the patient as a whole and avoid merely focusing on the skin or a minute aspect of it. A magnifying glass can be a useful tool, but a view of the doctor's face through the magnifying glass as he or she enters the room is probably no great comfort to the patient!

The examination should take place in a room with a good source of light, preferably daylight. A lesion of uncertain diagnosis when viewed in a dim light can become an obvious BCC, with pearly appearance and traversing telangiectasia, in a good light. In most cases the whole of the skin (or at least the vast majority of it) should be examined, with the patient wearing underclothes only. 'Window dermatology', a term originally used by me (CB Archer, 1995) to describe the situation when limited areas of the skin are offered and examined, is not good clinical practice and could be a dangerous practice, with consequent medicolegal implications. A good dermatologist will always consider the possibility of a concealed malignant melanoma and, for this reason along with the wish to provide a proper medical service to patients, will be reluctant to offer a dermatological opinion in the hospital corridor to even the most esteemed of medical colleagues.

The hair and nails are important skin appendages and the oral mucosa should be examined in many instances, if not routinely. The genital mucosal surfaces should be examined if indicated. Lichen planus is an example of a skin disease that commonly affects the buccal mucosa (sometimes other mucosal surfaces) and may be associated with nail dystrophy and scarring alopecia.

When examining the skin, it is usual to consider the form or morphology of individual lesions, the overall distribution on the body, and the pattern of the lesions in relation to each other. In practice (and with experience), these three assessments are made almost simultaneously and many skin disorders become instantly recognizable.

Morphology

Lesions may be solitary or multiple. A rash (or eruption) describes the complete picture of multiple lesions and its use should not be restricted to a description of a confluent red rash, as seen, for example, in measles. A maculopapular rash, strangely enough, consists of both macules and papules.

It is usual to describe the size, colour, consistency (is it soft or firm?), shape, margins (is there a sharp or diffuse edge?), and surface characteristics of skin lesions. For example, one might refer to a large brown rough-surfaced seborrhoeic keratosis, a small firm reddish dermatofibroma or a large soft lipoma with diffuse edge.

The shape of the lesions can point to the diagnosis. Annular lesions or plaques are commonly seen. Epidermal changes, such as scaling, crusting, excoriation, and lichenification, occur in psoriasis, discoid eczema, tinea corporis (ringworm), pityriasis rosea, lichen planus, and secondary syphilis. Granulomatous change in the dermis, giving rise to a slightly knobbly appearance of the skin, is seen in granuloma annulare, sarcoidosis, lupus vulgaris (a form of cutaneous tuberculosis), and leprosy. Erythema or oedema in the dermal layer is more likely to represent urticaria, erythema multiforme, or an annular erythema.

Distribution

Skin lesions may be localized or widespread. Although there will be many exceptions, several characteristic distributions exist and common skin disorders are often symmetical. A unilateral scaly annular rash may be due to a fungal infection.

In children and adults, atopic dermatitis tends to affect the antecubital and popliteal fossae, the periocular regions and nape of the neck, as well as other areas if severe. In infancy, atopic dermatitis affects the face and extensor aspects of the limbs, whereas flexural eczema at this age, with scalp involvement, is characteristic of seborrhoeic eczema (seborrhoeic dermatitis). The terms eczema and dermatitis are best used synonymously and there are several types (see Chapter 2).

Psoriasis characteristically involves the elbows, knees, extensor aspects of the limbs, and the scalp, particularly the scalp margins. Seborrhoeic dermatitis in adults usually affects the scalp, paranasal regions, eyebrows, and sometimes the presternal area, the interscapular skin, and flexures. Pityriasis rosea presents with red, scaly, oval plaques on the chest and back. There is usually a characteristic 'Christmas tree' arrangement of the lesions on the back and, with the exception of the upper thighs, the legs are largely spared.

Acne vulgaris occurs on the face, chest, and back, reflecting the distribution of the sebaceous glands, whereas acne rosacea is nearly always confined to the face, being a more common cause of a facial eruption of 'butterfly' distribution than the much-quoted rash of systemic lupus erythematosus.

In addition to the shape of individual lesions and their distribution, the **pattern** in which lesions are arranged may be characteristic. The two main patterns are linear and grouped lesions.

Linear lesions may be of developmental origin, as one sees with epidermal naevi, or determined by the Koebner or isomorphic phenomenon, in which skin lesions are localized to a site of injury such as a scratch or scar. This can occur in psoriasis, lichen planus, plane warts, or molluscum contagiosum warts. Herpes zoster (shingles) follows the distribution of a peripheral nerve, pain or tenderness frequently preceding the characteristic vesicular

Table 1.4 Skin disorders according to body regions

Region	Skin disorder
Face	Acne vulgaris
	Rosacea
	Facial eczema
	Seborrhoeic dermatitis
	Contact dermatitis
	(Atopic dermatitis)
	Lupus erythematosus
	(Psoriasis)
Trunk	Acne vulgaris
	Psoriasis
	Pityriasis rosea
	Pityriasis/tinea versicolor
	(Seborrhoeic dermatitis)
	Drug eruption
Limbs	Atopic dermatitis
	Psoriasis
	Discoid eczema
	Lichen planus
	(Varicose/venous eczema)
Hands and feet	Pompholyx
	Contact dermatitis
	Atopic dermatitis
	Psoriasis
	Tinea
	Scabies
Flexures	Tinea
	Psoriasis
	Seborrhoeic dermatitis
	Hidradenitis suppurativa
	Erythrasma
Scalp	Psoriasis
	Seborrhoeic dermatitis
	Tinea capitis
	Lupus erythematosus
	Lichen planus

eruption. Contact with exogenous materials is often linear, the linear blisters and streaky pigmentation of a phytophotodermatitis being a striking example. Grouped papules or nodules, particularly on the lower legs, should alert the physician to the possibility of insect bites.

Having emphasized the need to look at the patient as a whole, it can be useful to think of a differential diagnosis based on which region (or regions) of the body is involved (Table 1.4).

A good **clinical photography** service is desirable and, in some situations, the examination of previous photographs of lesions is an essential part of managing the patient (e.g. when looking for changes in a patient with multiple atypical naevi). There will be occasions when a general medical examination will be required and there is often the need to look for signs of anaemia, altered thyroid function (as in diffuse hair loss), lymphadenopathy, or hepatomegaly (e.g. in assessment of a patient with a skin tumour or lymphoma).

Clinical investigations

The clinical investigation of skin disorders will depend, to an extent, on the diagnostic acumen of the physician, and one should aim to carry out well-directed, relevant tests, thereby avoiding expensive and unnecessary investigations.

Dermatological investigations may include the need for histopathological examination of the skin; general laboratory investigations; allergy and photobiology tests; hair and nail investigations; bacteriology, mycology, and virology investigations; and tests for HIV-related and tropical skin infections.

A number of simple bedside investigations may confirm the clinical diagnosis. These include the use of dermatoscopy, a Wood's light, collection of skin scrapings and nail clippings for mycology (Chapter 12), dermographic testing, diascopy, the extraction of the acarus mite in scabies, and urine testing.

Dermatoscopy

Dermatoscopy involves the examination of the surface of pigmented lesions at moderate magnification using a dermatoscope, having first smeared the epidermis with gel or oil to prevent interference from reflected light. Interpretation of dermatoscopy findings requires training and experience, since it is important not to miss the diagnosis of a malignant melanoma.

One can see the distribution of melanin in the epidermis and superficial dermis in great detail.

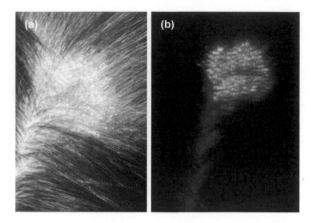

Figure 1.26a and b   Wood's light demonstration of tinea capitis, showing blue-green fluorescence.

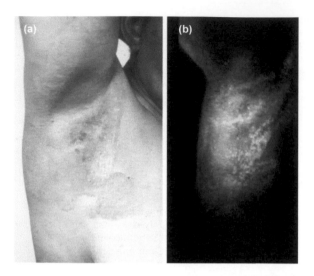

Figure 1.27a and b   Erythrasma, showing characteristic reddish-brown, slightly confluent areas in the right axilla and corresponding coral-red fluorescence under Wood's light.

Certain features are seen more commonly in malignant melanoma than in benign melanocytic naevi, but are not usually specific. These include peripherally situated black or brown dots and globules, a blue-white 'veil' appearance over the lesion, irregular pseudopods of pigment, and asymmetrical parallel linear extensions of pigment at the margin, known as 'radial streaming'. A lace-like melanin pigment network is found in both benign and malignant melanocytic lesions, but can be broadened and irregular in malignant melanoma.

Some non-melanocytic lesions have a characteristic appearance on dermatoscopy, including vascular lesions and BCCs. In acquired hemangiomas, small capillaries can be seen through the epidermis. BCCs often have a characteristic 'clover leaf' pattern of bluish pigmentation, which is due to dermal melanin or altered blood trapped within the BCC cell nests. Seborrheic keratoses have obvious keratin pits that can also be seen with the naked eye on the surface.

Wood's light

A Wood's light emits long-wave ultraviolet light in the 320–365 nm range of the spectrum. The light should be switched on a few minutes before use and the patient should be examined in a darkened room to allow any fluorescence to be seen.

In tinea capitis (Figure 1.26a and b), lesions due to *Microsporum canis* and *M. audouinii* show a brilliant blue-green fluorescence, whereas those due to *Trichophyton schoenleinii* fluoresce with a dull green colour. Erythrasma (Figure 1.27a and b), caused by *Corynebacterium minutissimum,* produces a characteristic coral-pink colour, usually in the axillae or groin region. Pityriasis versicolor may be detected by the observation of pale yellow fluorescence and the Wood's light may allow one to see lesions on the trunk that are not clinically apparent.

Wood's light can also be used to determine the depth of melanin in the skin. Variations in epidermal pigmentation are easier to see under Wood's light than in visible light (as in vitiligo or the ash-leaf macules of tuberous sclerosis). However, dermal pigmentation changes are less obvious under Wood's light (as in a blue naevus).

The 'acarus hunt'

Early on in my dermatology training, this endearing term conjured up images of the doctor searching for the scabies mite, armed with a monocle, shield, and spear! I have since discovered that a number of implements may be used to seek out the acarus, *Sarcoptes scabiei*. Careful exploration with a sterile needle of a scabies burrow, often in a finger web (see Chapter 12), may reveal the female mite clinging to the needle near the tip.

Even when a diagnosis of scabies is strongly suspected from the history, morphology, and distribution of the lesions, it is often difficult to find a linear burrow. The medial aspects of the feet may have been spared from excoriation. If no burrow is found, one may use a fine blade (a Gillette or scalpel blade) to perform a shave biopsy of a papule, ideally one which is not excoriated. A local anaesthetic is usually not required and the occurrence of pinpoint bleeding demonstrates the correct depth of the procedure. Several shave samples may be placed on a microscope slide, covered with immersion oil, and examined under low power. In this way, one may see a scabies mite, eggs, and faeces. Immersion oil is preferred to potassium hydroxide, since KOH dissolves the faeces.

Alternatively, application of immersion oil or KOH to an affected interdigital space, followed by light scraping with a scalpel blade, may reveal the beast and its eggs.

FURTHER READING

Archer CB. Clinical assessment of the dermatology patient. In: Cerio R, Archer CB (eds). Clinical Investigation of Skin Disorders. London: Chapman and Hall Medical, 1998.

Archer CB, Robertson SJ. Black and White Skin Diseases: an Atlas and Text. Oxford: Blackwell Science, 1995.

Bolognia JL, Jorrizzo JL, Rapini RP, et al. (eds). Dermatology. Philadelphia: Mosby, 2003.

Burns T, Breathnach S, Cox N, Griffiths C (eds). Rook's Textbook of Dermatology, 7th edn. Oxford: Blackwell Science, 2004.

Menzies S, Crotty K, Ingvar C, McCarthy WH. An Atlas of the Surface Microscopy of Pigmented Lesions, 2nd edn. Sydney: McGraw–Hill, 2003.

Stolz W, Braun Falco O, Bilek P, et al. Colour Atlas of Dermatoscopy, 2nd edn. Berlin: Blackwell Science, 2002.

CHAPTER 2

Disorders with epidermal change

PSORIASIS AND OTHER PAPULOSQUAMOUS
  DISEASES
Psoriasis
Other papulosqamous diseases
ECZEMA / DERMATITIS
Atopic dermatitis
Seborrhoeic dermatitis

Other endogenous eczemas
Contact dermatitis
OTHER INFLAMMATORY SKIN DISEASES
DISORDERS OF KERATINIZATION
The ichthyoses
Acantholytic diseases
Other disorders of keratinization

PSORIASIS AND OTHER PAPULOSQUAMOUS DISEASES

The papulosquamous disorders are characterized by the clinical appearance of scaling papules (e.g. lichen planus) and plaques (e.g. psoriasis, pityriasis rubra pilaris), in which, in contrast to the eczemas, the lesions are well-demarcated and not usually associated with crusting, excoriations, or weeping.

Psoriasis

Psoriasis is a common inflammatory, hyperproliferative papulosquamous disorder characterized by red scaly plaques. It affects about 2% of the population with equal sex incidence, occurs at any age (peak incidence 18–25 years old), and tends to run a chronic course. It has a multifactorial inheritance, often skipping generations, and has been associated with several HLA-specific antigens, particularly the HLA CW-6 antigen. The putative gene at *PSORS1*, the locus residing within the major histocompatibility complex (MHC) on the short arm of chromosome 6, is a major genetic determinant for psoriasis, thought to account for up to 50% of the heritability of the disease. There is much evidence that T lymphocytes have an important role in the development of psoriasis.

The most common pattern is chronic plaque psoriasis, usually affecting the elbows, knees, extensor aspects of the limbs, and the scalp. Other patterns include guttate (frequently following a streptococcal sore throat in young individuals), flexural (moist red patches), pustular (localized to the hands and feet or generalized), and erythrodermic psoriasis. In generalized pustular or erythrodermic psoriasis, sometimes occurring after erroneous administration of systemic corticosteroids, the patient may be very ill. Nail changes include pitting, thickening, onycholysis, and subungual hyperkeratosis, and in about 10% of cases there is an associated seronegative arthritis. Contrary to some earlier texts, patients with psoriasis do sometimes complain of itching.

In black skin, the redness and silvery scales of psoriasis are not usually seen, the predominant colour change being violaceous with overlying grey scaling. However, the distribution of the lesions, often accompanied by typical nail and scalp changes, usually makes the diagnosis quite easy. As in other skin diseases, psoriasis can sometimes take on a follicular appearance in black patients.

Guttate psoriasis often clears spontaneously, whereas plaque psoriasis is usually a chronic but treatable problem. There is a small mortality rate associated with generalized pustular or erythrodermic psoriasis, particularly in the elderly.

In most patients with psoriasis a skin biopsy is not required. It may sometimes be difficult to distinguish psoriasis from discoid eczema, and in this situation a biopsy usually shows features of psoriasis and eczema. The terms 'eczematous psoriasis' and 'psoriasiform eczema' are occasionally used, and the precise diagnosis will often become obvious as the skin disease evolves. It is wise to perform a skin biopsy in a patient with erythroderma, in case there are features of a lymphoma or drug eruption, common causes of erythroderma being psoriasis, atopic dermatitis (atopic eczema), and contact dermatitis.

In guttate psoriasis, a positive ASO titre or the more specific anti-DNase B titre may point to a streptococcal trigger for the rash, with a consequent low threshold in such patients for treating subsequent sore throats with penicillin. In the early stages, streptococci may be isolated from a throat swab. In an erythrodermic patient with lymphadenopathy, one should check the peripheral blood film for atypical mononuclear cells. Over 5% suggests Sézary syndrome (Chapter 6), whereas a lesser percentage is found in other patients with erythroderma.

Therapeutic suggestions
Vitamin D analogues
Topical corticosteroids
Topical corticosteroid/salicylic acid combination
Dithranol (anthralin)
Coal tar

Second-line treatment
UVB
Narrow-band UVB
PUVA
Methotrexate
Ciclosporin
Acitretin
Fumaric acid esters
Etanercept
Efalizumab
Infliximab

Other papulosqamous diseases

Pityriasis rubra pilaris (PRP) is a chronic papulosquamous disease in which there are familial and acquired forms. The lesions are reddish-brown follicular papules that coalesce to form confluent patches, which can involve most of the skin surface, with characteristic islands of sparing. The palms and soles show diffuse hyperkeratosis.

Therapeutic suggestions
Acitretin

Second-line treatment
Oral methotrexate

Seborrhoeic dermatitis and superficial fungal diseases fulfil the clinical description of papulosquamous diseases, as do lichen planus and pityriasis rosea, which are considered also as disorders of the dermal–epidermal interface and the dermis (Chapter 4).

ECZEMA / DERMATITIS

These terms are often used synonymously, as in this book. In the USA the term dermatitis is used non-specifically to mean 'an inflammatory skin disease'. I prefer the more specific usage of dermatitis as a less cumbersome way of saying 'eczematous dermatitis', and it is not necessary to retain the previous habit in the UK of relating the terms eczema and dermatitis to endogenous and exogenous causes, respectively.

There are several types of eczema, characterized by the clinical appearance of itchy, red, scaly skin, sometimes with vesicles (the clinical manifestation of epidermal oedema or 'spongiosis'), exudation, and crusting. These include atopic dermatitis (atopic eczema), seborrhoeic dermatitis, discoid eczema, pompholyx, varicose eczema, asteatotic eczema, primary irritant and allergic contact dermatitis. Sometimes eczema may be predominantly due to endogenous or exogenous factors, but the aetiology of eczema is often multifactorial. As in other fields of medicine, it is desirable to be as specific about the diagnosis as possible, and a diagnosis of atopic dermatitis, for example, is much more specific than the general term 'eczema', although this may be a useful term in epidemiological studies.

Atopic dermatitis

Atopic dermatitis (synonymous with atopic eczema) is usually defined as an itchy chronic or chronically relapsing, inflammatory skin disease. The rash is characterized by itchy papules (occasionally vesicles), which become excoriated and thickened, and typically have a flexural distribution. Atopic dermatitis occurs in up to 25% of children, the onset of the disease being in the first year of life in 60%, and is frequently seen in patients with a personal or family history of atopic diseases (i.e. asthma, allergic rhinitis, or atopic dermatitis). The importance of genetic factors in determining the expression of the atopic phenotype has been shown in twin studies. Genetic linkage studies have identified a number of genes related to the expression of different atopic syndromes, immunoglobulin E (IgE) levels, and cytokines relevant to the regulation of IgE levels, but no causal gene has yet been identified for atopic dermatitis. A number of cell regulatory abnormalities in mononuclear leukocytes (monocytes and lymphocytes) have been reported in atopic dermatitis, which may, in turn, lead to an exaggerated response of the skin to trigger factors in the environment, such as irritants (e.g. detergents, house dust) and antigens (e.g. cow's milk, house dust mite).

In atopic dermatitis the skin is often dry and extremely itchy. Scratching makes the eczema worse and produces lichenification. The severity fluctuates with time and secondary bacterial infection, usually with *Staphylococcus aureus*, can be recognized by exudation and crusting. Any part of the body can be affected, often symmetrically. In infancy, the face and extensor aspects of the limbs are usually involved, whereas in older children and adults the eczema tends to affect the flexures (e.g. antecubital and popliteal fossae), the periocular regions, and the nape of the neck.

In black skin, close inspection of the skin may reveal erythema with epidermal changes, such as scaling, and the distribution of the eruption may be as in white skin. However, the predominant colour changes are often those of post-inflammatory hyperpigmentation or, less commonly, hypopigmentation and the elbows, knees, and extensor aspects of the limbs can be involved in the so-called 'reverse pattern' of atopic dermatitis. The lesions can also be accentuated around hair follicles (follicular eczema). Excoriation associated with itching and impetigonization from secondary bacterial infection are also useful signs.

In any patient with itching, one should also look carefully for the linear burrows of scabies, since the reaction of the skin to this is eczematous. **Pityriasis alba** is commonly seen on the cheeks of black children in the presence or absence of atopic dermatitis.

Skin and nasal swabs (before antibiotic therapy) can help direct treatment, particularly in atopic dermatitis. Patients with atopic dermatitis usually have raised serum IgE levels with multiple positive skin prick test or radioallergosorbent test (RAST) responses to common antigens. However, these tests are not performed routinely, since they are of limited diagnostic use, and patients (or their parents) may overinterpret the significance of an individual positive result, assuming, for example, that the eczema is 'caused' by the house dust mite, which may be one of many trigger factors. A skin biopsy is not usually required.

Atopic dermatitis improves with age: around 50% of those presenting in infancy resolve by the age of 10 years old.

Therapeutic suggestions
Emollients
Topical corticosteroids
Topical immunosuppressive agents (calcineurin inhibitors)
Antihistamines (usually sedative)
Topical and oral antibiotics

Second-line treatment
Oral corticosteroids
Azathioprine
Ciclosporin
UVB
PUVA
Mycophenolate mofetil

Seborrhoeic dermatitis

Seborrhoeic dermatitis is common, and yeasts on the skin play an important causative role in predisposed individuals. Endogenous and exogenous factors therefore play a role in the aetiology and pathogenesis. In infancy, seborrhoeic dermatitis affects the scalp and flexures (napkin dermatitis), frequently allowing the distinction from atopic dermatitis. Features of seborrhoeic dermatitis in adults include dandruff, paranasal and eyebrow scaling, and sometimes eczema in the presternal, interscapular, axillary, and groin regions. Seborrhoeic dermatitis is usually responsive to therapy but tends to recur if treatment is stopped.

Therapeutic suggestions
Topical miconazole plus hydrocortisone
Topical ketoconazole
Topical hydrocortisone

Second-line treatment
Itraconazole

Other endogenous eczemas

The circular lesions of **discoid (nummular) eczema** usually occur on the extensor aspects of the limbs in adults but may be widespread. In **pompholyx (cheiropompholyx)**, patients often have large painful blisters on the palms and soles, with smaller itchy vesicles along the sides of the fingers. In the elderly, **varicose (venous) eczema** is common, affecting the lower legs and sometimes accompanied by venous ulcers. **Asteatotic eczema (eczema craquelé)**, associated with drying of the skin (e.g. following admission to hospital) usually affects the shins and the scaling takes on a 'crazy paving' appearance. Discoid eczema and asteatotic eczema are frequently seen in the same patient. The tendency to develop discoid eczema and pompholyx often resolves over a period of 2 years, whereas varicose eczema usually persists.

Contact dermatitis

Exogenous factors can worsen all types of eczema and may be causative in **primary irritant** or **allergic contact dermatitis**, the latter being a cell-mediated immune (type IV) response. Common sensitizers include nickel (as in costume jewellery), chromium, rubber, medicaments (including topical neomycin and preservatives), plants and pre-polymerized plastics and glues in industry.

Contact dermatitis often involves the hands where it can be difficult to be sure of the aetiology based on the pattern of eczema alone. However, primary irritant dermatitis may initially involve the finger webs and the flexor aspects of the wrists, where the epidermis is thinner than on the palms.

Patch testing to a standard battery of allergens and sometimes other potential sensitizers will often confirm a clinical diagnosis of allergic contact dermatitis. The distinction between allergic and irritant responses can be difficult and, to minimize false-positive results, patch tests should be performed in a specialist dermatology department. An **open or usage test** is a helpful adjunct to patch testing. The patient applies the agent twice daily to the skin inferior to the antecubital fossa. Production of eczema indicates the relevance of the allergen. No reaction after 2–3 days shows that any positive patch test reaction was a false-positive result.

Contact dermatitis can resolve completely on avoidance of exogenous factors, although this may not be so for certain sensitizers (e.g. chromate in cement workers).

Specialist investigation of eczema*

Tests of immediate hypersensitivity:

  Skin prick tests

  Intradermal tests

  Scratch tests

  IgE and RASTs

Patch testing

Open or usage tests

Photopatch testing

*These investigations require careful selection and interpretation in the context of the clinical situation.

OTHER INFLAMMATORY SKIN DISEASES

Included in this group of disorders are **chronic actinic dermatitis, exfoliative dermatitis, perioral dermatitis, juvenile plantar dermatosis** (often occurring in atopics), **lichen simplex chronicus,** nodular prurigo, and **lichen striatus. Dermatitis artefacta** can be induced in a variety of ways.

Nodular prurigo is an intensely itchy dermatosis in which lichenified nodules develop on the arms, shins, and upper back. There is an increased incidence of iron deficiency and atopy in patients with nodular prurigo, and there is marked post-inflammatory hyperpigmentation in black skin.

Therapeutic suggestions

Topical corticosteroids

Topical corticosteroids with polythene occlusion

Capsaicin

Second-line treatment

UVB

PUVA

Thalidomide

The differential diagnosis of eczema/dermatitis includes psoriasis, pityriasis rosea, fungal infections (which are often unilateral), drug eruptions, disseminate and recurrent infundibulo-folliculitis, and infantile acropustulosis.

Disseminate and recurrent infundibulo-folliculitis (described by Hitch and Lund) is an extremely itchy, often persistent, follicular eruption that occurs almost exclusively in patients with black skin. **Infantile acropustulosis** is more common in black skin and presents with pruritic vesicles or pustules primarily on the hands and feet of infants. There is little response to topical corticosteroids or antibiotics, but the disorder resolves spontaneously after 2–3 years.

DISORDERS OF KERATINIZATION

These diseases include the ichthyoses, Darier's disease, keratosis pilaris, and the many forms of palmoplantar keratoderma.

The ichthyoses

The ichthyoses are a group of disorders in which there is generalized persistent scaling of the skin. The process is non-inflammatory, although some forms of ichthyosis are accompanied by erythema. The term **ichthyosis vulgaris** refers to an autosomal dominant disorder, affecting about 1 in 250 children, in which the extensor aspects of the skin are characteristically involved and patients have hyperlinear palms.

X-linked recessive ichthyosis affects male offspring who inherit an X chromosome bearing a steroid sulphatase genetic mutation from their asymptomatic mother, leading to steroid sulphatase deficiency. Affected boys have distinctive larger brown scales and the flexures also tend to be involved. Steroid sulphatase enzyme activity can be measured in leukocytes or skin fibroblasts, and is much reduced or absent in X-linked recessive icthyosis.

Bullous ichthyosiform erythroderma (BIE, epidermolytic hyperkeratosis) is a rare autosominal dominant disease presenting shortly after birth, the erythema and blistering decreasing as the child grows older. **Non-bullous ichthyosiform erythroderma** (NBIE) is an uncommon recessive disease in which affected infants have generalized erythroderma and fine scaling of the entire skin surface. **Lamellar ichthyosis**, a rare recessive disease, has been distinguished from NBIE by the presence of generalized thick hyperkeratotic scaling and the relative lack of erythema. Ichthyosis also forms part of a number of syndromes (e.g. Refsum's syndrome, Netherton's syndrome) and, as with other ichthyoses, the biochemical abnormalities underlying these diseases are now better understood.

Collodion baby or lamellar desquamation of the newborn are terms used synonymously to describe a characteristic clinical entitiy which may be a reflection of several distinct clinical varieties of ichthyosis. In most cases collodion baby is the initial manifestation of NBIE (or lamellar ichthyosis).

Harlequin fetus is a very rare congenital, often fatal abnormality in which there is a hard fissured hyperkeratotic covering to the skin, with ectropion, abnormalities of the lips, and small deformed (or absent) ears.

Acantholytic diseases

Acantholysis refers to loss of coherence between epidermal cells and characteristically occurs in pemphigus vulgaris in which there are initially clefts and then bullae in a predominant suprabasal location, and Hailey–Hailey disease (Chapter 5). The acantholytic diseases considered here are Darier's disease and Grover's disease.

Darier's disease (keratosis follicularis) is an uncommon autosomal dominant disorder in which patients have greasy brown keratotic papules on the forehead, face, neck, and upper trunk, macerated intertriginous lesions, and characteristic nail changes, with longitudinal ridges, distal notching, and red and white linear subungual bands. Sun exposure often exacerbates the disease and secondary bacterial infection is common.

Therapeutic suggestions
Emollients
Topical retinoids

Second-line treatment
Acitretin

Grover's disease (transient and persistent acantholytic dermatosis) presents as an acute eruption of pruritic papules or papulovesicles, mainly affecting the trunk, and is more common in men than women. Heat and sweating are predisposing factors and its relationship to Darier's disease is debatable.

Therapeutic suggestions
Emollients
Avoid heat and sweating
Topical corticosteroids

Other disorders of keratinization

Keratosis pilaris is the commonest type of follicular keratosis and is characterized by keratinous plugs in follicular orifices, with varying degrees of perifollicular erythema. Occasionally, keratosis pilaris is succeeded by atrophic skin changes, as seen in **keratosis pilaris atrophicans faciei** or **ulerythema ophryogenes**, in which the process is mainly confined to the eyebrow region. Keratosis spinulosa (lichen spinulosus) is a clinical variant of keratosis pilaris.

Therapeutic suggestions
Emollients
Topical retinoids
Topical tazarotene

Kyrle's disease (hyperkeratosis follicularis et parafollicularis) and **Flegel's disease** (hyperkeratosis lenticularis perstans) are uncommon disorders of keratinization.

The histologically distinct **porokeratoses** are sub-classified into 3 autosomal dominant types: porokeratosis of Mibelli (with solitary or multiple linear lesions on the body), disseminated superficial actinic porokeratosis (often on the lower legs), and a porokeratosis that predominantly affects the palms and soles.

There are a number of types of **palmoplantar keratodermas**, including hereditary forms and those associated with other recognized diseases such as **pachyonychia congenita** and pityriasis rubra pilaris (PRP). Diffuse palmoplantar keratoderma is an autosomal dominant disorder and rare families have been described in which keratoderma (tylosis) has been associated with carcinoma of the oesophagus.

Included here is **acrokeratoelastoides**, which overlaps clinically to some extent with focal acral hyperkeratosis. **Focal acral hyperkeratosis** is a form of papular keratoderma that occurs almost exclusively in black Africans. It is characterized by oval papules, which may have central pigmented pits, situated on the borders of the palms and soles.

FURTHER READING

Bolognia JL, Jorrizzo JL, Rapini RP, et al (eds). Dermatology. Philadelphia: Mosby, 2003.

Burns T, Breathnach S, Cox N, Griffiths C (eds). Rook's Textbook of Dermatology, 7th edn. Oxford: Blackwell Science, 2004.

Lebwohl MG, Heymann WR, Berth-Jones J, Coulson I (eds). Treatment of Skin Disease: Comprehensive Therapeutic Strategies, 2nd edn. Philadelphia: Mosby Elsevier, 2006.

Murphy GM. Investigation of allergic skin disorders and the photodermatoses. In: Cerio R, Archer CB (eds). Clinical Investigation of Skin Disorders. London: Chapman and Hall Medical, 1998.

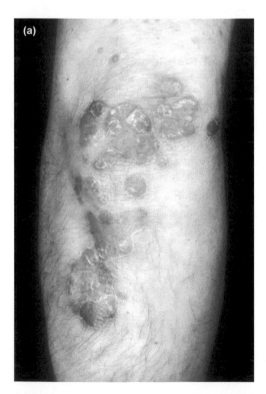
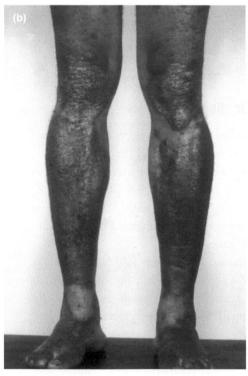

Figure 2.1a and b   Psoriasis, with erythematous inflammatory plaques on the elbow region (2.1a) and grey hyperkeratotic plaques on the knees, shins, and feet of a man of Indian origin (2.1b).

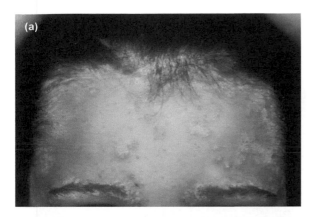

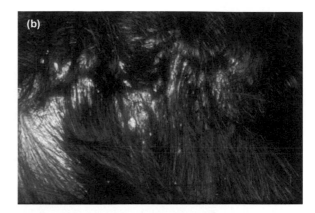

Figure 2.2a and b   (2.2a) Psoriasis affecting the hair margin and eyebrows. (2.2b) Pityriasis amiantacea in a patient with psoriasis. This clinical sign, in which hyperkeratotic scale remains attached to the growing hair, is also seen in seborrhoeic dermatitis.

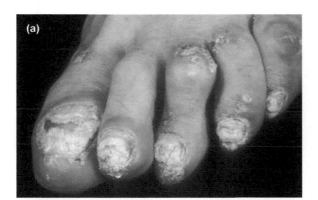

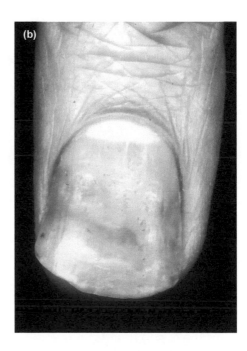

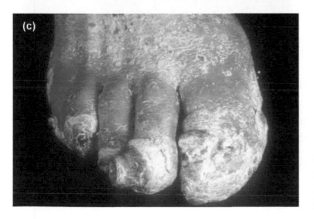

Figure 2.3a, b, and c   Psoriatic nail dystrophy. Nail changes in psoriasis include thickening, subungual hyperkeratosis (2.3a), onycholysis, and pitting (2.3b). (2.3c) Severe onychogryphosis in a patient with psoriasis.

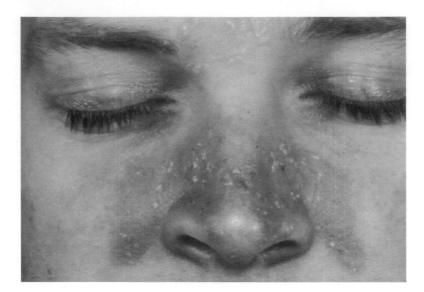

Figure 2.4   Facial psoriasis, with prominent paranasal involvement. This pattern of psoriasis can be difficult to distinguish from seborrhoeic dermatitis, but there are usually typical psoriatic lesions on other areas of the skin.

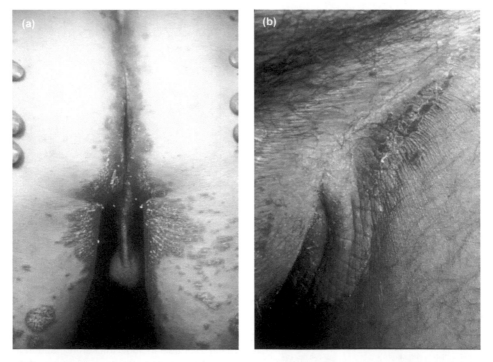

Figure 2.5a and b   Flexural psoriasis. (2.5a) Sore, red, shiny psoriasis affecting the natal cleft and groin region, with hyper-keratotic plaques on the thighs. (2.5b) Fissuring and grey scaling of the groin in an Indian man, with typical psoriasis elsewhere.

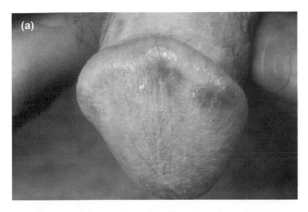
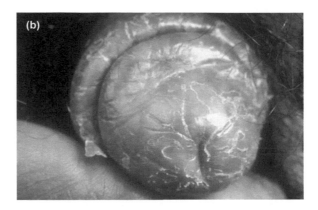

Figure 2.6a and b   Psoriasis affecting the glans penis. (2.6a) Pink, slightly scaly lesions and (2.6b) diffuse scaling of the glans penis, with post-inflammatory hyperpigmentation.

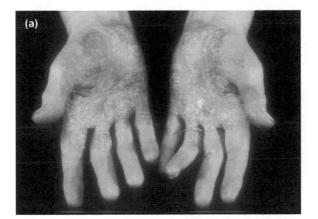
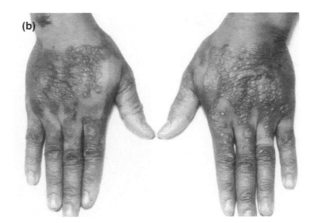

Figure 2.7a and b   Psoriasis on the hands. Palmar psoriasis can be difficult to distinguish from chronic hand eczema, but the absence of itchy vesicles is a helpful sign. (2.7a) Confluent hyperkeratotic erythematous psoriasis on the palms. (2.7b) In black skin, the violaceous colour with overlying grey scale is characteristic.

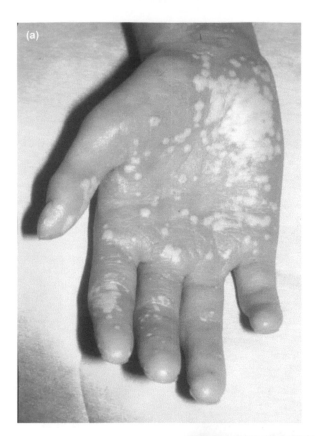

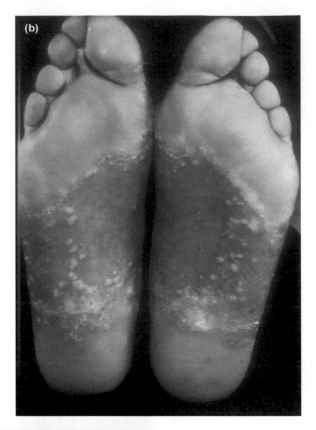

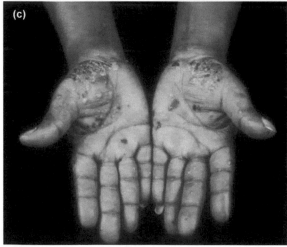

Figure 2.8a, b, and c   Localized pustular psoriasis. The sterile neutrophil-rich pustules are often confined to the palms (2.8a) and soles (2.8b). (2.8c) Localized pustular psoriasis of the palms in black skin. In the absence of psoriasis elsewhere, the term palmoplantar pustulosis is used. Patients with palmoplantar pustulosis tend to be cigarette smokers and the disease usually runs a chronic course.

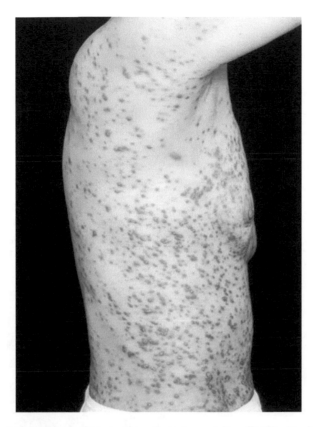

Figure 2.9   Generalized pustular psoriasis. Sheets of small sterile pustules affect the trunk and limbs, often with a background of confluent erythema. The onset is acute and the patient is frequently ill, with fever, malaise, and a leukocytosis. Generalized pustular psoriasis may be life-threatening, particularly in elderly patients.

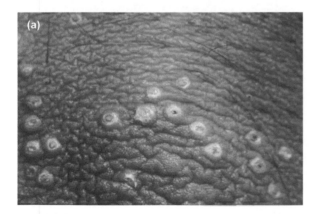

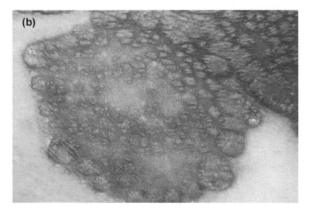

Figure 2.10a and b   (2.10a) In black skin psoriasis may be predominantly perifollicular. (2.10b) The typical short-lived epidermal brown staining caused by anthralin (dithranol) treatment in a patient with white skin.

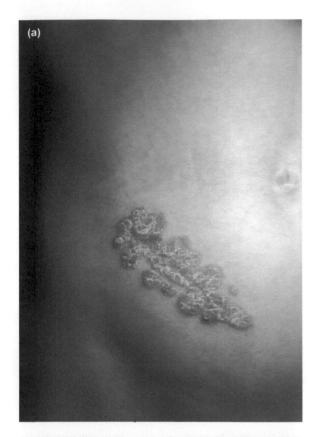

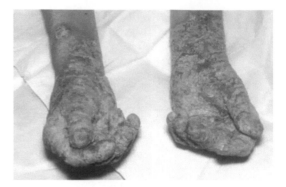

Figure 2.12   Psoriasis: acrodermatitis continua. This is an uncommon variant of psoriasis in which there is a severe inflammatory reaction affecting the hands and/or feet, sometimes with lakes of sterile pus adjacent to the nails.

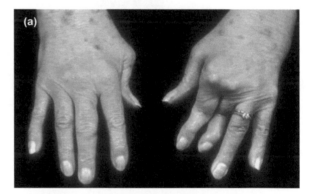

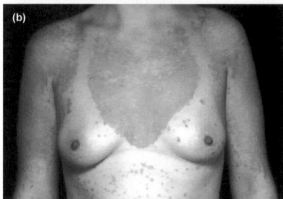

Figure 2.11a and b   Koebner (isomorphic) phenomenon in psoriasis. Psoriasis can localize to the site of injury to the skin, resulting from, for example, a scratch, burn (2.11a) or surgical trauma. (2.11b) The Koebner phenomenon occurs in psoriasis due to sunburn, although moderate sun exposure usually improves psoriasis. The Koebner phenomenon occurs in some, but not all, patients with psoriasis.

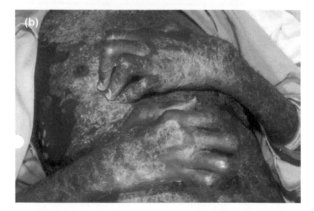

Figure   2.13a and b   Psoriatic arthropathy. A seronegative arthritis occurs in about 10% of patients with psoriasis. Various types include a distal arthropathy (in contrast to rheumatoid arthritis, usually involving the terminal interphalangeal joints of the hands), a monoarthritis (e.g. of the knee or hip joint), ankylosis of the vertebral column, and a severe arthritis of the hands, sometimes resembling rheumatoid arthritis.

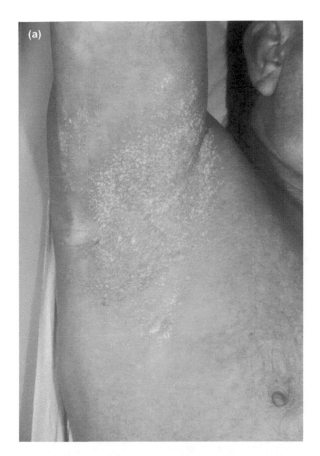
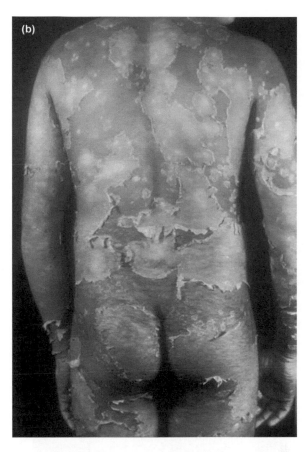

Figure 2.14a and b Erythrodermic psoriasis. This may occur in a patient with known psoriasis or de novo, when the distinction from erythroderma associated with eczema/dermatitis, a drug eruption, or lymphoma may be difficult. Withdrawal of systemic corticosteroids can lead to erythrodermic psoriasis (2.14a) which may progress to generalized pustular psoriasis. With resolution of the process, the skin passes through a phase of desquamation (2.14b).

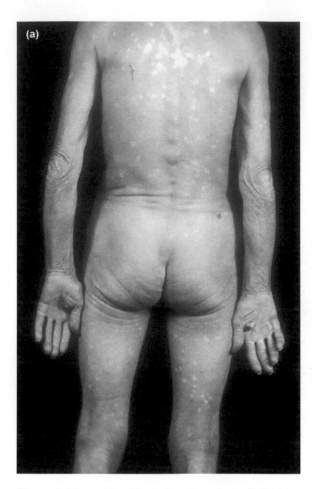 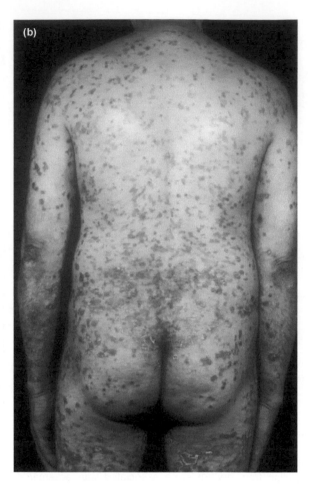

Figure 2.15a and b   Pityriasis rubra pilaris. (2.15a) Large areas of perifollicular papules on the trunk and limbs, with plaques on the elbows and hyperkeratosis of the palms. Characteristic islands of normal skin are seen on the upper back. (2.15b) Numerous psoriasis-like plaques and post-inflammatory hyperpigmentation.

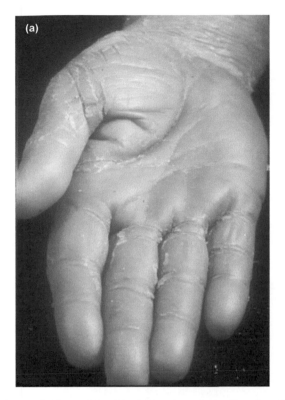

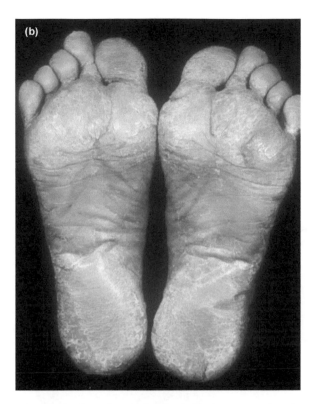

Figure 2.16a and b   Pityriasis rubra pilaris, showing diffuse palmoplantar hyperkeratosis. The typical orange colour is seen on the palmar skin (2.16a).

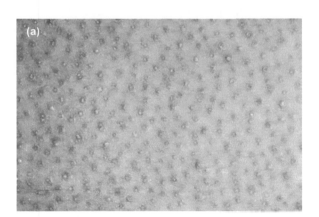

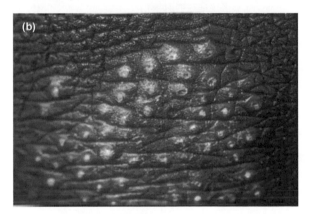

Figure 2.17a and b   (2.17a) Pityriasis rubra pilaris, showing the perifollicular inflammatory papules in white skin. (2.17b) In black skin, the inflammatory erythema may not be seen, but the follicular distribution of the lesions and post-inflammatory hyperpigmentation are readily visible.

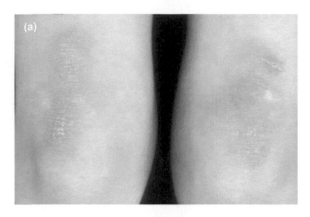

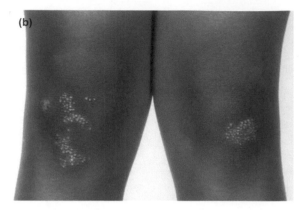

Figure 2.18a and b   Juvenile pityriasis rubra pilaris. The knees are commonly involved in affected children and the symmetrical nature of the disorder is apparent.

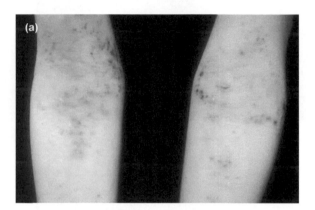

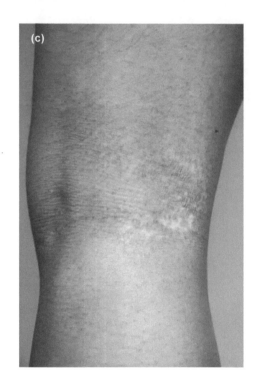

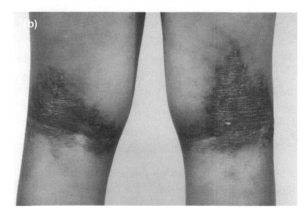

Figure 2.19a, b, and c   Atopic dermatitis. (2.19a) Excoriated lesions affecting the antecubital fossae. (2.19b and c) Views of the popliteal fossae, showing lichenification, post-inflammatory hyperpigmentation, and hypopigmentation associated with atopic dermatitis in deeply pigmented skin.

(a)

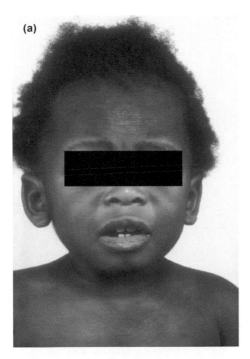

(b)

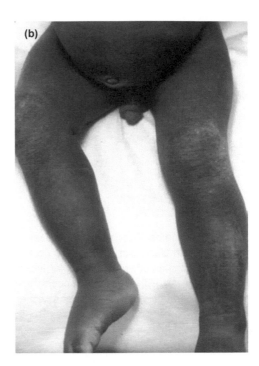

Figure 2.20a and b   Atopic dermatitis of infancy, with lichenified eczema and prominent hyperpigmentation on the forehead and upper chest (2.20a) and characteristic extensor involvement (2.20b) in an infant of West Indian origin.

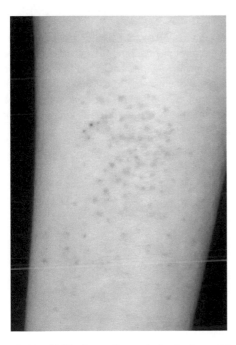

Figure 2.21   Follicular pattern of atopic dermatitis. The eczematous lesions are accentuated around hair follicles, as shown on the arm. This pattern more commonly occurs in deeply pigmented skin (see Chapter 1).

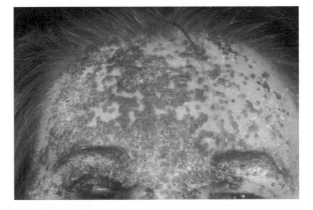

Figure 2.22   Eczema herpeticum. Superimposed infection with herpes simplex virus in patients with atopic dermatitis produces eczema herpeticum. The excoriated vesicular lesions are monomorphic in appearance and in severe cases, herpes encephalitis may ensue. Secondary bacterial infection, as shown here, is relatively common.

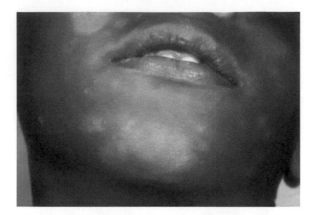

Figure 2.23   Pityriasis alba. This is commonly seen on the face in patients with black skin but can also occur in white patients. Hypopigmented, oval, or circular lesions are usually slightly scaly. Pityriasis alba occurs more commonly in atopic dermatitis patients but does occur in children without evidence of eczema, the differential diagnosis including post-inflammatory hypopigmentation.

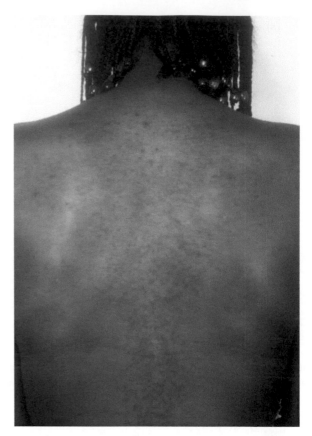

Figure 2.25   Pityrosporum folliculitis. As in seborrhoeic dermatitis, the role of pityrosporum yeasts was confirmed by the use of specific systemic antifungal agents. The follicular eruption is monomorphic. In black skin the predominant colour change is one of hyperpigmentation as opposed to erythema in white skin. The differential diagnosis includes follicular eczema and trichostasis spinulosa.

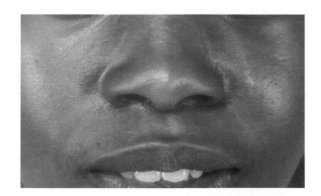

Figure 2.24   Seborrhoeic dermatitis. Erythema and scaling usually affect the paranasal regions. Patients usually have dandruff and the red, scaly rash may also affect the eyebrow, presternal, interscapular, and flexural regions. An element of rosacea frequently accompanies seborrheic dermatitis, when there might also be a history of papules, pustules, or flushing.

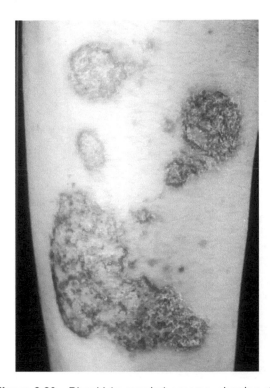

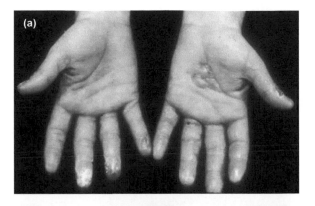

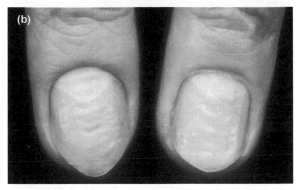

Figure 2.26   Discoid (nummular) eczema, showing circular, crusted lesions on the arm. This very itchy, persistent eczema tends to affect middle-aged men. Secondary bacterial infection is common. Discoid eczema responds to appropriate therapy but often recurs before subsiding after 1–2 years.

Figure 2.27a and b   Endogenous hand and foot eczema (cheiropompholyx), showing large, painful blisters on the palms (2.27a). There are often smaller itchy vesicular lesions along the sides of the fingers. (2.27b) The characteristic horizontal bands, seen in nail dystrophy associated with eczema of the nail fold region. Constitutional hand eczema may occur alone but is often accompanied by dermatitis affecting the soles of the feet.

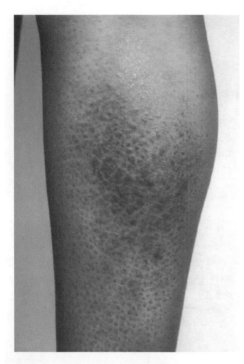

Figure 2.28   Asteatotic eczema (eczema craquelé), showing the typical 'crazy paving' appearance on the shins. This particularly affects elderly people when the skin is allowed to dry out excessively (e.g. during a hospital admission). The eczema readily responds to the use of emollients.

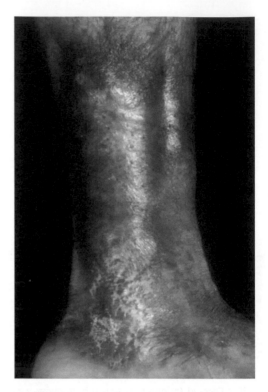

Figure 2.29   Varicose eczema, with post-inflammatory hyperpigmentation and some white areas of 'atrophie blanche'. Varicose eczema is often associated with venous ulcers.

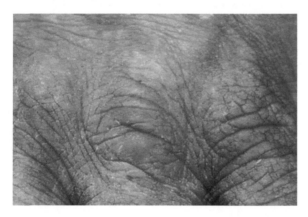

Figure 2.30   Primary irritant dermatitis, affecting the hands. This frequently follows the repeated immersion of the hands in detergents, such as washing up liquid (housewives' dermatitis). Initially the finger webs and anterior wrists are involved, sites where the epidermis is thinner than on the palms. However, any area of the skin on the hands may be affected. Detergents sometimes accumulate beneath a ring, leading to the false assumption that the patient has become allergic to the constituent metal.

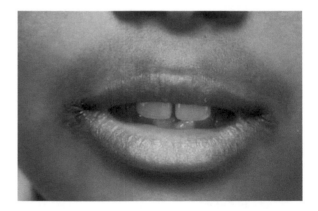

Figure 2.31   Lip licker's dermatitis. This is a form of irritant dermatitis commonly occurring in children as a result of licking the lips and surrounding skin. Adults tend to moisten one lip with the other. It can sometimes be difficult to break this habit and in black people the post-inflammatory pigmentary changes may persist for some time.

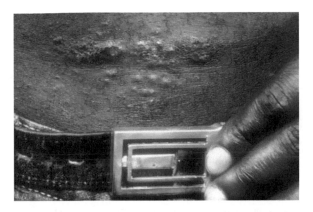

Figure 2.32   Allergic contact dermatitis from nickel in a belt buckle. Nickel dermatitis is common, affecting about 10% of women; other offending articles are costume jewellery (earrings, necklaces) and denim jean studs. In black people, the redness of the eczema may not be discernible but there is often scaly, itchy hyperpigmentation at the site of contact with metals.

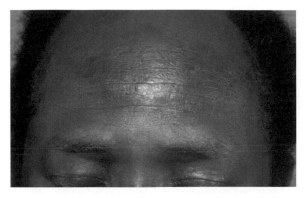

Figure 2.34   Allergic contact dermatitis from clothing, showing an eczematous reaction to chromate, contained in a leather hat band. Chromate dermatitis is also seen on the hands of cement workers, and on the feet due to leather shoes. Dermatitis of the feet also occurs from contact with rubber chemicals in footwear, the eruption particularly affecting the pressure points on the soles of the feet.

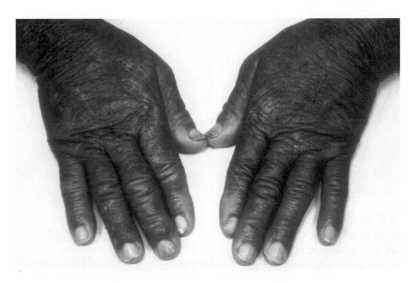

Figure 2.33   Allergic contact dermatitis from rubber. There is often a sharp cut-off line where the gloves have been in contact with the skin of the hands and forearms. The predominant change in black skin is that of post-inflammatory hyperpigmentation. The aetiology of hand eczema is often multifactorial with endogenous (e.g. atopic dermatitis), irritant, and allergic factors playing a part.

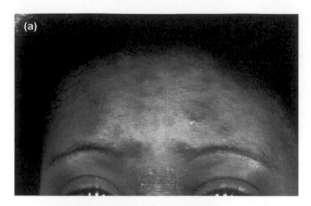

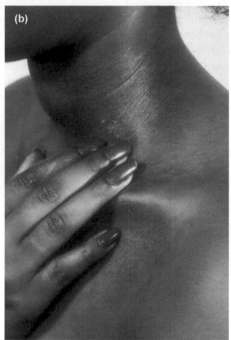

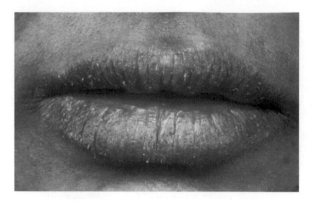

Figure 2.36 Lipstick dermatitis. The eczematous process is confined to where the lipstick has been applied, there being little perioral involvement, in contrast to lip licker's dermatitis. Allergic contact dermatitis from cosmetics and make-ups is a frequent cause of facial eczema and should be distinguished from facial involvement in atopic dermatitis or seborrhoeic dermatitis.

Figure 2.35a and b Nail varnish dermatitis. The eczema commonly affects the eyelids, the cheeks, and anterior and lateral aspects of the neck, the finger-tips being unaffected. In deeply pigmented skin there is often post-inflammatory hyperpigmentation and the pruritus and distribution of the eczema provide useful diagnostic clues. When patch testing, the nail varnish should be allowed to dry before applying the Finn chamber, in order to avoid false-positive irritant reactions.

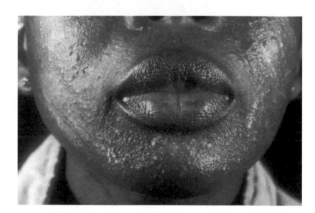

Figure 2.37 Allergic contact dermatitis from medicaments, showing an allergic contact dermatitis due to the application of an antifungal cream in a patient with black skin. The commonest situations in which this occurs is in the treatment of otitis externa and varicose eczema with venous ulceration. Common sensitizers include neomycin and sulphur-containing antibiotics.

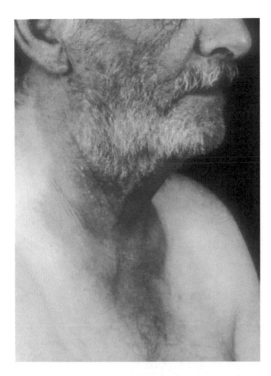

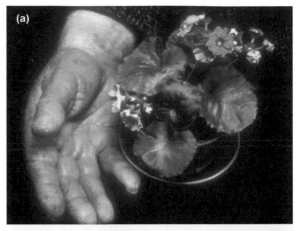

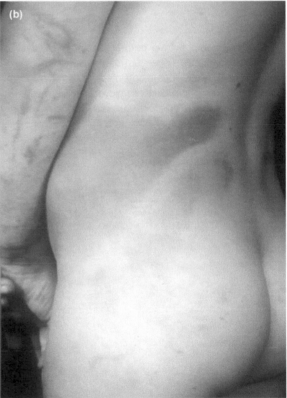

Figure 2.38 Allergic contact dermatitis from phosphorus sesquisulphide, found in red-tipped matches. The eczema commonly has an apparent photosensitive distribution, sometimes with an eczematous reaction affecting the skin underlying the pocket in which the patient keeps the box of matches. This form of dermatitis is now relatively uncommon due to the use of lighters and safety matches.

Figure 2.39a and b Plant dermatitis. (2.39a) An allergic eczematous reaction to *Primula obconica*. An acute streaky vesicular dermatitis commonly involves the forearm skin and the face. The other species of primula rarely cause an allergic contact dermatitis. In the USA, common sensitizers include poison oak and poison ivy. (2.39b) A phytophotodermatitis, a phototoxic reaction due to contact with psoralen-containing plants, such as rue. Characteristic linear lesions occur at the sites of contact, sometimes comprising large bullae and often resulting in prominent post-inflammatory hyperpigmentation.

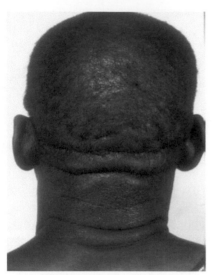

Figure 2.40 Chronic actinic dermatitis (photosensitive eczema). This represents a spectrum of disease severity in which photosensitivity develops in patients with other forms of long-standing eczema, including allergic contact dermatitis and atopic dermatitis. Multiple positive patch test reactions are often seen and the diagnosis may be confirmed by mono-chromator light testing. Although more common in white people, chronic actinic dermatitis does occur in black patients.

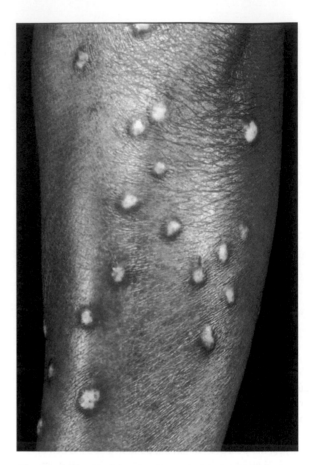

Figure 2.42 Nodular prurigo, showing marked post-inflammatory hyperpigmentation and excoriated nodules on the lower leg. The arms, legs, and upper back are usually involved in this intensely itchy dermatosis. There is an increased incidence of iron deficiency and atopy in patients with nodular prurigo.

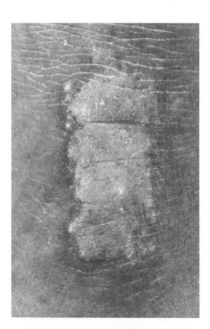

Figure 2.41 Lichen simplex chronicus, showing a thick-ened, lichenified lesion on the lower leg. This is a com-mon site for this chronic eczematous process in which the repeated act of scratching plays a major role. In black skin the lesions often have a silvery grey appearance, accompanied by post-inflammatory hyperpigmentation.

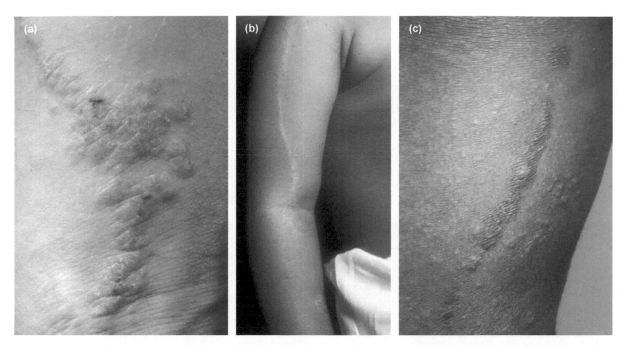

Figure 2.43a, b, and c Lichen striatus. This is a linear inflammatory disorder, often occurring on the limbs, the histology of which shows chronic eczematous changes. (2.43a) The similarity to chronic eczema. (2.43b and c) The post-inflammatory hypopigmentation or hyperpigmentation that may be seen in black skin. Lichen striatus usually reaches its full extent within a few weeks and resolves spontaneously over the next few months. The history distinguishes lichen striatus from linear epidermal naevi.

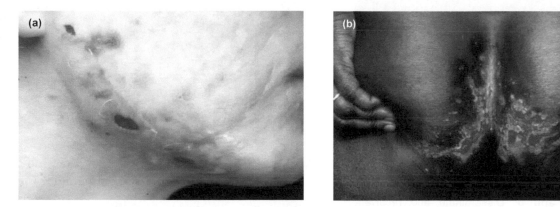

Figure 2.44a and b Dermatitis artefacta, showing bizarre exogenous-looking lesions. The face is a common site (2.44a) and the frequently linear lesions may be produced in a variety of ways: e.g. with a sharp instrument or by the application of a caustic solution. Other body sites may be involved (2.44b), the latter showing ulceration on the buttocks and hyperpigmentation in previously active sites. Psychologically disturbed patients are also sometimes rather adept at imitating recognized diseases such as the porphyrias.

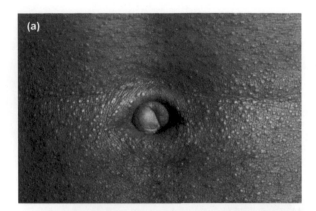

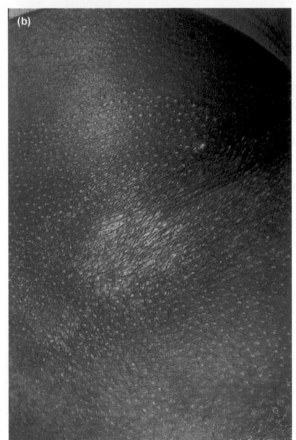

Figure 2.45a and b Disseminate and recurrent infundibulo-folliculitis, showing monomorphic extremely itchy perifollicular lesions on the trunk and thigh of a man of Afro-Caribbean origin. This disorder occurs almost exclusively in blacks and is often very persistent, failing to respond to topical corticosteroids and emollients. The histology shows spongiosis of the outer part of the hair follicles and the main differential diagnosis is that of follicular eczema.

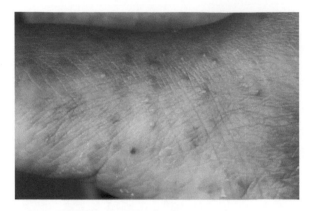

Figure 2.46 Infantile acropustulosis, showing itchy reddish vesicles on the foot of a young child. This disorder is more commonly seen in black skin.

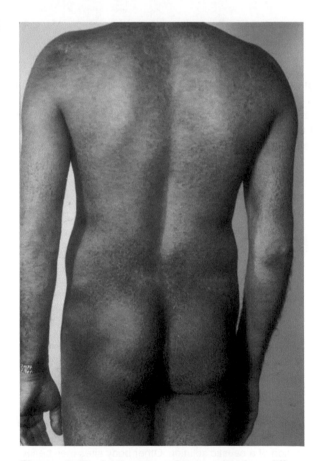

Figure 2.47 Ichthyosis vulgaris, showing diffuse ichthyotic changes on the trunk and buttocks. Although ichthyosis is a non-inflammatory disease, in black skin there may be prominent hyperpigmentation. Sometimes this may be due to associated atopic dermatitis.

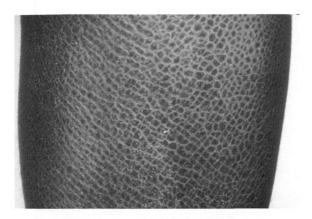

Figure 2.48   X-linked ichthyosis. Compared with autosomal dominant ichthyosis vulgaris, affected boys have larger brown scales and the flexures are usually involved. The dark brown colour of the individual scales is seen, separated by a lighter background pigmentation in a patient of Afro-Caribbean origin.

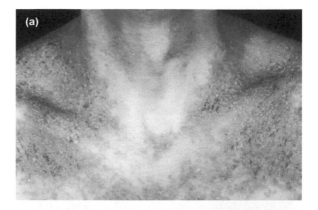

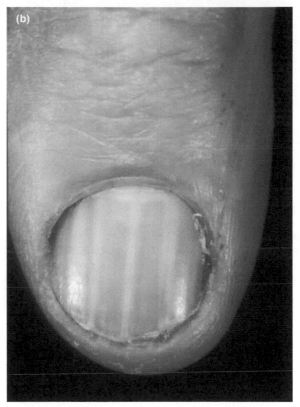

Figure 2.49a and b   Darier's disease (keratosis follicularis), showing confluent reddish hyperkeratotic and erosions, reflecting epidermal acantholysis, on the upper trunk (2.49a). Secondary bacterial infection plays a role in this disease, which is exacerbated by sun exposure. (2.49b) The characteristic red and white linear subungual bands and distal notching of a finger nail.

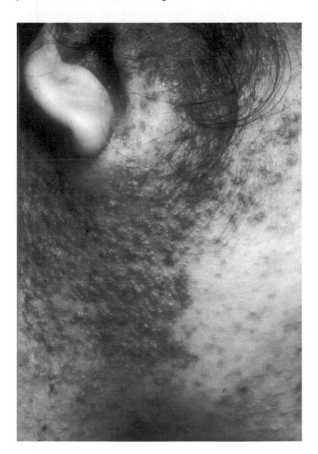

Figure 2.50   Darier's disease (keratosis follicularis). The scalp margins and face are commonly involved with greasy, brown, keratotic papules.

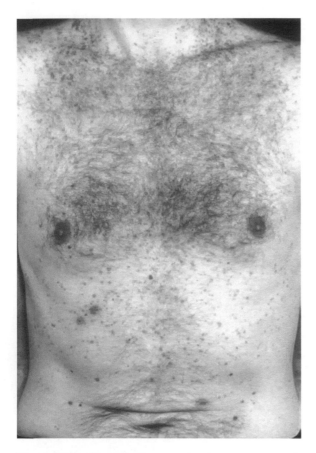

Figure 2.51   Grover's disease, showing numerous reddish itchy lesions on the trunk. This eruption is often provoked by sun exposure and can involve the face and neck, in addition to the trunk. The diagnosis is confirmed by the finding of epidermal acantholysis on histology. (Courtesy of Dr HA Fawcett.)

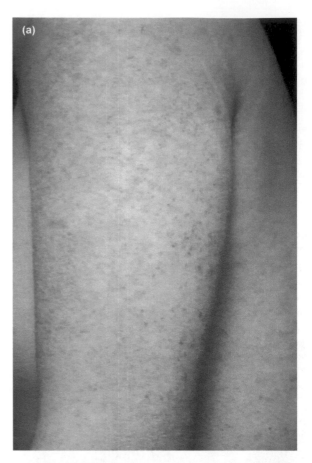

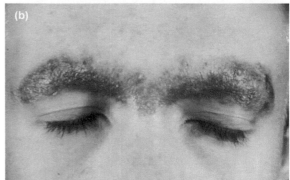

Figure 2.52a and b   Keratosis pilaris (2.52a), showing keratotic papules on the upper arms. KP is a common finding in patients of Mediterranean origin. It is occasionally associated with atrophic changes in the eyebrow region (2.52b), referred to as keratosis pilaris atrophicans faciei (ulerythema ophryogenes).

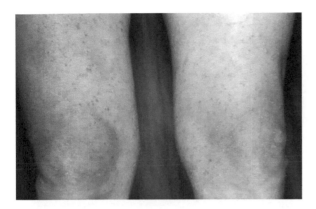

Figure 2.53 Kyrle's disease (hyperkeratosis follicularis et parafollicularis), showing hyperkeratotic plaques on the thighs and knees.

(a)

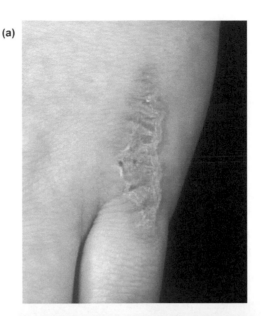

(b)

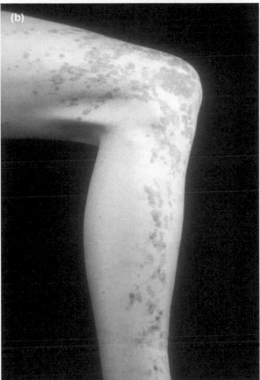

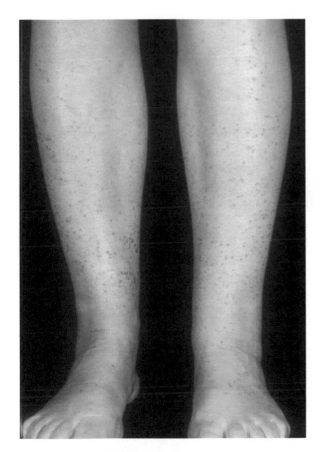

Figure 2.54 Flegel's disease (hyperkeratosis lenticularis perstans), showing red, rather persistent keratotic lesions on the lower legs. The differential diagnosis includes the other disorders of keratinization, Kyrle's disease, and disseminated superficial actinic porokeratosis.

Figure 2.55a and b Porokeratosis, a group of autosomal dominant disorders. (2.55a and b) The linear keratotic lesions of porokeratosis of Mibelli, which may be solitary or multiple. The lesions of disseminated superficial actinic porokeratosis (DSAP) predominantly affect the lower legs of middle-aged or elderly women.

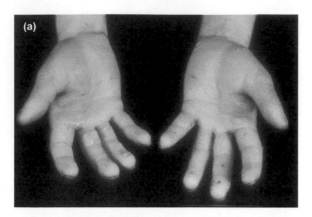
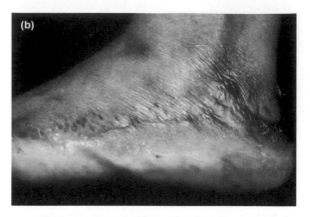

Figure 2.56a and b   Palmoplantar keratoderma, showing diffuse hyperkeratosis of the palms (2.56a) and keratoderma extending onto the sides of the foot, with hyperpigmentation in a man of Afro-Caribbean origin (2.56b).

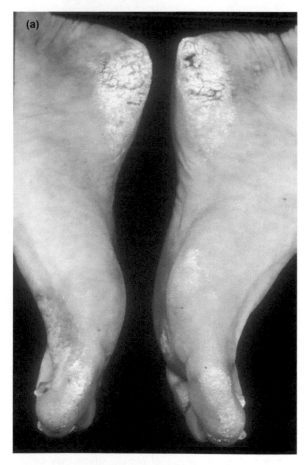
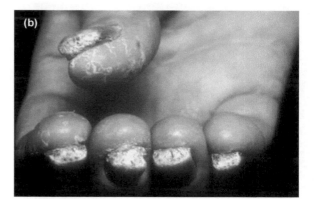
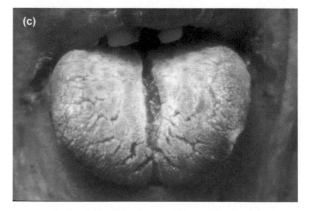

Figure 2.57a, b, and c   Pachyonychia congenita, showing localized areas of hyperkeratosis on the soles (2.57a) with the characteristic wedge-shaped nail changes, here shown on the hands (2.57b). Some patients with pachyonychia congenita have leukoplakia on the tongue (2.57c).

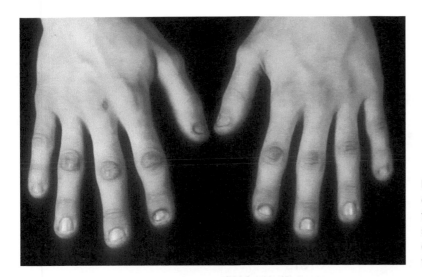

Figure 2.58 Knuckle pads, showing circumscribed fibromatous lesions over the finger joints. Knuckle pads may occur sporadically or may be familial. Trauma does not seem to be a significant factor in the aetiology.

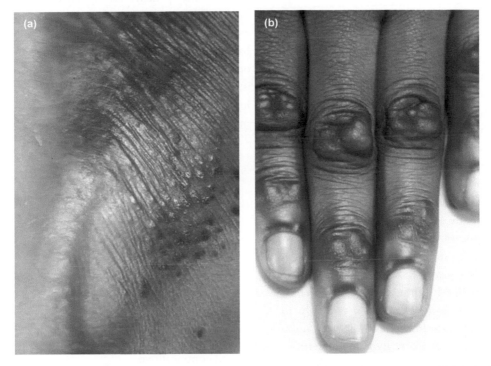

Figure 2.59a and b Acrokeratoelastoides, showing firm warty papules on the ankle in a patient with black skin (2.59a). The pearly papular lesions are usually seen on the sides of the hands, fingers, and wrists. Lesions resembling knuckle pads may also occur as seen in the same patient (2.59b) and hyperpigmentation is a common feature. Clinically, the disorder overlaps to some extent with focal acral hyperkeratosis, the histology of which shows no reduction in the number of dermal elastic fibres.

CHAPTER 3

Disorders of the epidermal appendages and related disorders

ACNE
ROSACEA AND PERIORAL DERMATITIS
PSEUDOFOLLICULITIS BARBAE
HIDRADENITIS SUPPURATIVA

FOX–FORDYCE DISEASE
CYSTS
HAIR PROBLEMS

ACNE

Acne vulgaris is a common disorder of the pilosebaceous units, affecting up to 90% of adolescents, in which hyperactivity of sebaceous glands leads to increased sebum production (seborrhoea or greasy skin) with hypercornification of the pilosebaceous duct. Adolescents may present with blackheads (open comedones) in which the colour is due to melanin pigmentation, whiteheads (closed comedones), papules, pustules, nodules, cysts, and varying degrees of scarring, usually on the face, chest, and back.

The differential diagnosis includes rosacea (in which blackheads are absent), perioral dermatitis (as induced by application of a fluorinated corticosteroid to the face), milia (small epidermal cysts), sarcoidosis, or plane warts.

In deeply pigmented skin it is important to commence treatment as early as possible, not only to prevent scarring but also to avoid unnecessary, often persistent post-inflammatory hyperpigmentation. Pomade acne is commonly seen on the forehead of black patients who apply oils and greasy creams to the hair.

Patients with severe nodulocystic acne or persistent acne despite other treatments may require treatment with oral isotretinoin. As part of the monitoring process, such patients usually have baseline fasting lipids and routine liver function tests which are repeated after 1 month (and again only if indicated). A baseline pregnancy test at the appropriate time is recommended in females of child-bearing potential and it is essential for such patients not to become pregnant for the usual 4–6-month course of isotretinoin or for a month either side of the treatment.

Therapeutic suggestions
Topical benzoyl peroxide
Topical antibiotics
Topical retinoids
Azelaic acid
Oral antibiotics (e.g. oxytetracycline, lymecycline, minocycline)

Second-line treatment
Combined antiandrogen and oestrogen oral contraceptive
Oral isotretinoin

Acne keloidalis nuchae is a disease which is nearly always seen in black men, usually during their late teens. Firm papules develop on the nape of the neck or in the hair-bearing occipital region and later coalesce to form keloidal bands with scarring alopecia. In chronic cases there may be pustules and subcutaneous abscesses with draining sinuses. Acne keloidalis can be very difficult to treat, but promising results have been reported following excision down to the fascia or deep subcutaneous tissue and healing by secondary intention.

Therapeutic suggestions
Oral antibiotics
Intralesional corticosteroids

Second-line treatment
Excision down to fascia, allowing to heal by secondary intention

Keloids due to acne on the trunk, particularly on the chest and posterior shoulders, also occur in white patients and are often multiple.

ROSACEA AND PERIORAL DERMATITIS

Rosacea usually occurs in patients between 30 and 50 years of age, and is commoner in women than men. Intermittent flushing of the cheeks, nose, forehead, and chin is triggered by being in a hot room, alcohol, spicy foods, and, in some, exposure to sunlight. The redness may become persistent, with telangiectasia, papules, pustules, and lymphoedema. The absence of blackheads in acne rosacea helps to distinguish the disorder from acne vulgaris, although there are patients who have features of both. Rhinophyma (enlargement of the nose, usually in men) may occur and ocular effects include blepharitis, conjunctivitis, and keratitis. Rosacea can occur in deeply pigmented skin but is claimed to be rare in patients of Afro-American origin.

Therapeutic suggestions
Topical metronidazole
Oral antibiotics

Second-line treatment
Topical tretinoin
Azelaic acid
Topical sulphur
Oral isotretinoin

The differential diagnosis includes **perioral dermatitis**, which is often associated with the repeated application of a topical fluorinated corticosteroid. Perioral dermatitis may also complicate rosacea if a fluorinated corticosteroid has been used in error.

Therapeutic suggestions
Withdrawal of topical fluorinated corticosteroids
Oral tetracyclines

PSEUDOFOLLICULITIS BARBAE

Pseudofolliculitis barbae is relatively common in men of Afro-Caribbean or African origin. Shaving of the stiff, curved hairs produces a sharp tip, which then tend to grow laterally, penetrating the skin of the beard area to set up a foreign body reaction, resulting in papules, pustules, and sometimes prominent post-inflammatory hyperpigmentation. The best way to cure the disease is to stop shaving, but such advice is not always accepted by the patient. The beard should not be shaved too short and patients are sometimes recommended to use a small brush (e.g. a toothbrush) to brush the hairs away from the skin. There may be an accompanying folliculitis of the beard area, which may require treatment, usually with a topical antibiotic or a low dose of a tetracycline.

Therapeutic suggestions
Beard growth
Razor shaving technique

Second-line treatment
Topical or oral antibiotics

Other facial appendageal disorders include the comedones, follicular cysts, and prominent elastosis of the **Favre–Racouchot syndrome**, seen in men with chronic sun damage, **milia** (sometimes occurring in infancy), and **syringomas** (**hidrocystomas**), derived from sweat glands.

HIDRADENITIS SUPPURATIVA

Hidradenitis suppurativa is a chronic, deep-seated inflammatory scarring disease of the apocrine glands in the axillae and groins. An early event in the pathological process is the comedonal occlusion of the apocrine glands as they open into the pilosebaceous ducts, obstructing the outflow of the apocrine glands and sebaceous glands. The process is probably androgen-driven and secondary bacterial infection is thought to lead to the tender inflamed lesions, with pustules, abscesses, and scarring of the dermis. Hidradenitis begins after puberty and affects women more commonly than men. Women with hidradenitis do not have an increased incidence of acne. Occasionally hidradenitis can be part of the '**follicular occlusion triad**', in which patients also have acne conglobata and a perifolliculitis of the scalp.

Therapeutic suggestions
Oral antibiotics
Intralesional corticosteroids

Second-line treatment
Oral isotretinoin

FOX–FORDYCE DISEASE

Fox–Fordyce disease is a disorder of the apocrine glands, occurring mainly in females and beginning during puberty. Patients initially present with itching in the axillae, on the breasts, and sometimes in the perineum. Obstruction of the sweat duct with keratin is associated with the development of reddish dome-shaped follicular papules and, in black patients, hyperpigmentation.

Therapeutic suggestions
Topical corticosteroids
Intralesional corticosteroids

Second-line treatment
Electrodesiccation

CYSTS

The term 'sebaceous cyst' is frequently used as a general term for cysts in the skin, although cysts which are derived from sebaceous glands are uncommon. Commonly encountered cysts include **epidermal (epidermoid) cysts** and **pilar (trichilemmal) cysts**, the latter being derived from hair follicles and occurring predominantly on the scalp. **Steatocystoma multiplex (sebocystomatosis)**, in which there are multiple cysts in the dermis, the walls of which contain sebaceous gland lobules (i.e. these are true sebaceous cysts), is rare and sometimes inherited as an autosomal dominant condition.

HAIR PROBLEMS

Hair problems may be considered as hair loss (alopecia), excessive hair growth (hirsutism and hypertrichosis), or as abnormalities of the hair shaft.

There are a number of different types of alopecia, which can be identified by the pattern of hair loss, a careful history regarding other medical illnesses, and the patient's habits. There is a group of scarring forms of alopecia, and the presence of scarring, which can be difficult to be sure of clinically, is an important diagnostic feature.

Alopecia areata is usually easily recognized in white or black patients, and may be associated with a personal or family history of other autoimmune diseases such as vitiligo, thyroiditis, pernicious anaemia, and diabetes mellitus. The severity of the process may vary, but in most cases the hair regrows over a period of 1–2 years.

An autoimmune profile may show positive thyroid or gastric parietal cell antibodies, but measurement of these antibodies does not affect the management of the patient.

Therapeutic suggestions
Topical corticosteroids
Topical minoxidil

Second-line treatment
Intralesional corticosteroids
Topical diphencyprone
Oral corticosteroids

Male pattern hair loss is very common and there is a **female pattern**, in which hair thinning occurs as opposed to baldness. An androgenic pattern of hair loss merits measurement of sex hormone-binding globulin and plasma testosterone. When these are abnormal, further investigation is required to exclude polycystic ovarian syndrome (PCOS).

Diffuse alopecia is relatively common, particularly in women. Iron deficiency is an important cause of hair loss in women. Thyroid function tests may reveal hypothyroidism or, more rarely, hyperthyroidism. Alopecia areata can present with diffuse hair loss.

Scarring alopecia may be part of inflammatory diseases such as cutaneous discoid lupus erythematosus (CDLE) and lichen planopilaris, a form of lichen planus. Frontal fibrosing alopecia seems to be related to lichen planopilaris and is sometimes seen in patients with evidence of lichen planus elsewhere.

Folliculitis decalvans is a scarring alopecia which results from a chronic pustular folliculitis of the scalp, sometimes involving *Staphylococcus aureus*. Tufted folliculitis is a variant of folliculitis decalvans in which circumscribed areas of scalp inflammation heal, with scarring characterized by tufts of several hairs emerging from a single orifice.

Therapeutic suggestions
Topical antibiotics

Second-line treatment
Oral antibiotics (e.g. clindamycin and rifampicin)

The occurrence of **traumatic alopecia** often depends on hair fashions, and at present this type of hair loss, including traction alopecia, 'hot comb alopecia', and alopecia associated with other hair-grooming techniques, is more common in black patients. The term 'central centrifugal alopecia' has been used as an alternative to hot comb alopecia. Not all women with central centrifugal alopecia will have used hot combs but the attachment of brades to their hair makes the situation worse.

Trichotillomania occurs as a result of pulling, twisting, and/or rubbing the hair. Mild trichotillomania is quite common in children, but there are sometimes serious underlying psychological problems which may persist into adulthood.

Alopecia neoplastica is a rare form of hair loss in which metastases of the scalp appear as scleroderma-like plaques. Metastatic deposits in the scalp more commonly present as dermal nodules that may erode the epidermis.

Hirsutism describes excessive hair growth in an androgen-dependent pattern in females. As this disorder merges with normality, endocrine investigations are often normal, in part reflecting different end-organ responses to normal circulating androgens. Hirsutism associated with acne and oligomenorrhoea may be a presenting feature of PCOS.

Typically, the ratio of plasma luteinizing hormone (LH) to follicle-stimulating hormone (FSH) is increased, and testosterone, oestradiol, and androstenedione levels are raised.

> **Therapeutic suggestions**
> Hair removal (e.g. laser, electrolysis)
> Eflornithine
>
> **Second-line treatment**
> Oral contraceptives
> Metformin
> Spironolactone

Hirsuties may be associated with hyperprolactinaemia or, in childhood, with congenital adrenal hyperplasia. The affected child usually has other features of virilization and altered electrolyte status due to salt loss.

Generalized hypertrichosis (non-androgenic excessive hair growth) may be seen in Cushing's syndrome, in which the plasma cortisol levels will be elevated, and hypothyroidism in children. Hypertrichosis of light-exposed skin occurs in some cases of erythropoietic protoporphyria and almost all of the rarer porphyrias, congenital erythropoietic porphyria, and porphyria variegata. It is also seen on the trunk and limbs in mucopolysaccharidoses such as Hurler's syndrome.

Abnormalities of the hair shaft may be associated with increased fragility, as in **pili torti** (twisting of hair), for example, or may not be associated with increased fragility, as one sees in **pili annulati** (ringed hair). Increased fragility presents clinically as patchy or diffuse alopecia.

FURTHER READING

Bolognia JL, Jorrizzo JL, Rapini RP, et al (eds). Dermatology. Philadelphia: Mosby, 2003.

Burns T, Breathnach S, Cox N, Griffiths C (eds). Rook's Textbook of Dermatology, 7th edn. Oxford: Blackwell Science, 2004.

Lovell CR. General laboratory investigations. In: Cerio R, Archer CB (eds). Clinical Investigation of Skin Disorders. London: Chapman and Hall Medical, 1998.

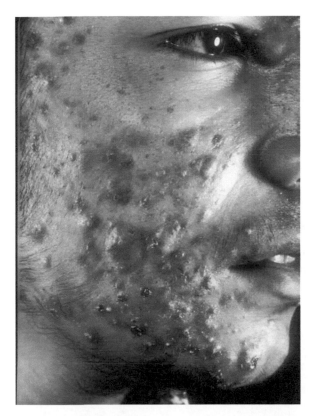

Figure 3.1 Acne vulgaris, showing papules, pustules, and nodulocystic lesions on the face. Facial lesions are seen in most cases, the chest and back being involved in about 70% of cases.

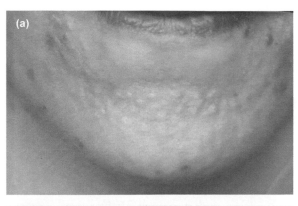

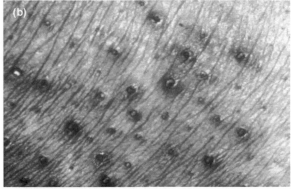

Figure 3.2a and b Acne vulgaris, showing (3.2a) whiteheads (closed comedones) and (3.2b) blackheads (open comedones).

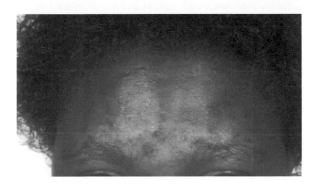

Figure 3.3 Acne vulgaris. In black skin, post-inflammatory hyperpigmentation is often prominent and may persist long after the active disease process has resolved. Forehead lesions are commonly seen in black patients following the regular application of oils and greasy materials to the hair (pomade acne).

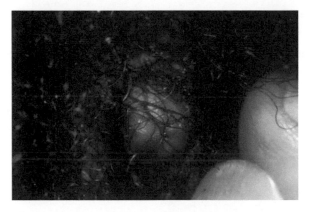

Figure 3.4 Acne keloidalis nuchae, showing a characteristic keloidal lesion on the occipital region in a black patient. Initially, firm papules develop on the nape of the neck and occipital region, later leading to keloidal bands with scarring alopecia. This disorder nearly always affects black men but white people are occasionally affected.

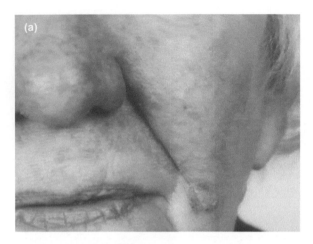

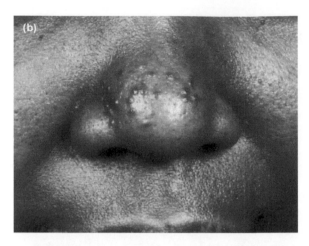

Figure 3.5a and b   Acne rosacea, showing redness, telangiectasia and papules on the nose and cheeks in an elderly white woman (3.5a). In black skin, the erythema is not apparent and papules and pustules predominate, as seen on the nose (3.5b).

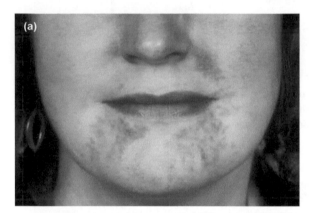

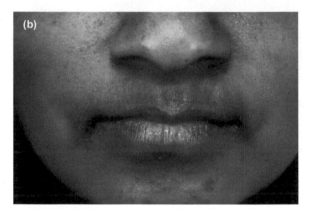

Figure 3.6a and b   Perioral dermatitis, showing papules and pustules in the perioral region (3.6a). The application of fluorinated corticosteroids to facial skin is a frequent cause. (3.6b) Post-inflammatory hyperpigmentation in deeply pigmented skin.

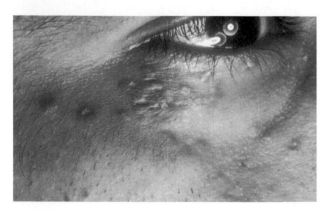

Figure 3.7   Acne agminata (lupus miliaris faciei), showing reddish-brown lesions inferior to the right lower eyelid in an Indian patient. This is a granulomatous disorder in which the histology may resemble granulomatous rosacea.

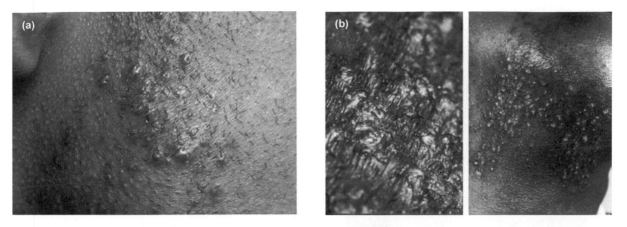

Figure 3.8a and b   Pseudofolliculitis barbae, with multiple firm papules on the cheek and neck, due to a foreign body reaction to penetrating hairs. (3.8a and b) Varying degrees of post-inflammatory hyperpigmentation. This disorder can sometimes be difficult to distinguish from keloid formation in black males with active acne vulgaris.

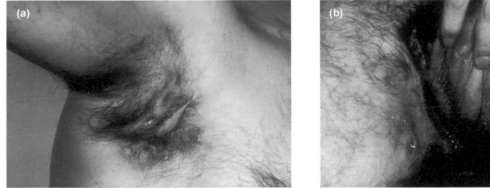
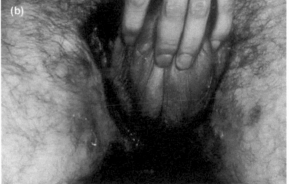

Figure 3.9a and b   Hidradenitis suppurativa, showing deep-seated scarring inflammatory lesions in the axilla (3.9a) and groin region (3.9b). This man also had acne conglobata, and perifolliculitis of the scalp (the follicular occlusion triad).

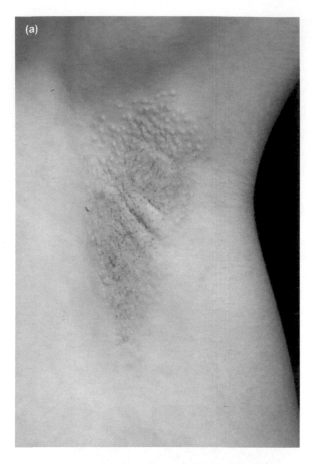

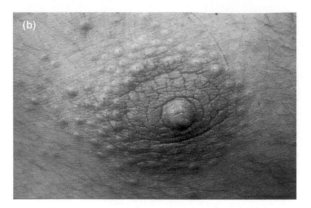

Figure 3.10a and b Fox–Fordyce disease, showing papular lesions in the axilla (3.10a) and adjacent to the areola in an Indian patient (3.10b). The papular lesions are derived from apocrine glands.

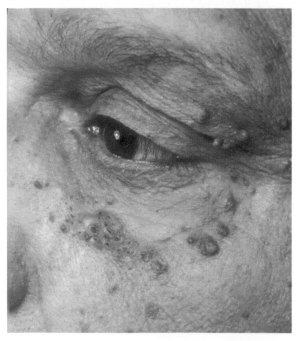

Figure 3.11 The Favre–Rachouchot syndrome. Large comedones are seen in elderly people and are often associated with sun-induced elastotic changes. The triad of large (giant) comedones, prominent elastosis, and follicular cysts is referred to as the Favre–Rachouchot syndrome.

(a)
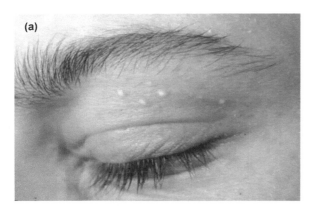

(b)
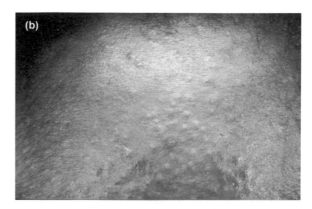

Figure 3.12a and b   Milia. These white thin-walled epidermal cysts are common, occurring as solitary or multiple lesions on the face.

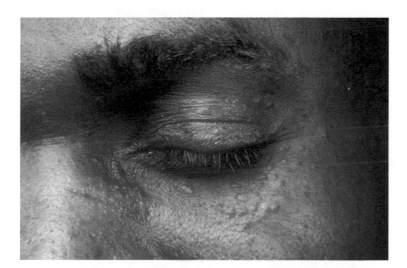

Figure 3.13   Syringomas (hidrocystadenomas), showing characteristic papules in the periocular region. Syringomas are benign sweat duct tumours which are usually multiple.

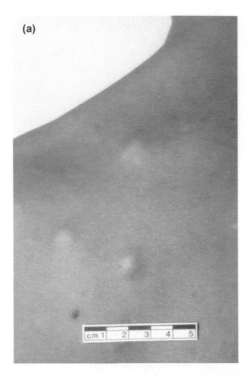

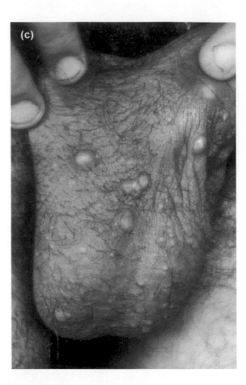

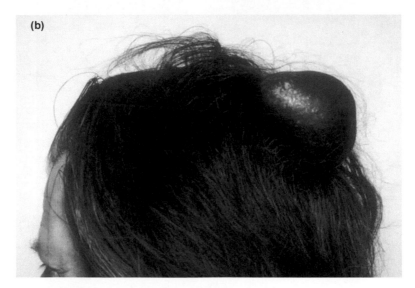

Figure 3.14a, b, and c   Epidermoid cysts, often incorrectly referred to as sebaceous cysts, have an epidermal cell lining and contain keratin. They commonly occur on the trunk (3.14a). A pilar or trichilemmal cyst is derived from the hair follicle and is seen on the scalp or on other hair-bearing areas, such as the eyebrow and scalp (3.14b). Cysts also occur in severe acne and, uncommonly, as multiple lesions on the scrotum (3.14c).

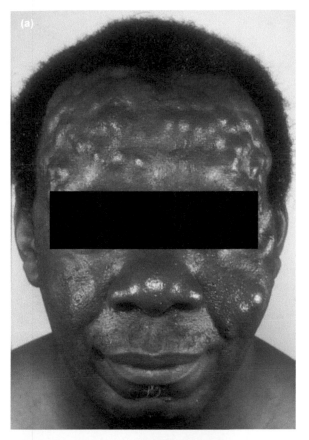

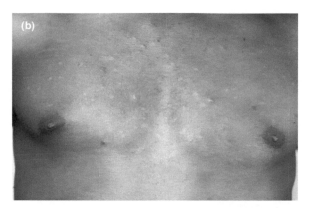

Figure 3.15a and b Steatocystoma multiplex. This is an uncommon disorder in which there are multiple cysts in the dermis, each with sebaceous gland lobules in the cyst wall and containing sebum (i.e. they are true sebaceous cysts). They can occur on the face (3.15a), but the trunk (3.15b) and proximal part of the limbs are more commonly involved.

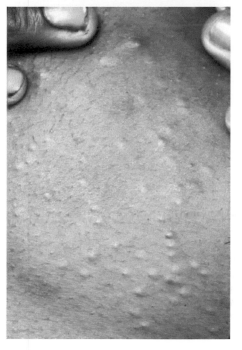

Figure 3.16 Eruptive vellus hair cysts are asymptomatic follicular papules, 1–2 mm in size, usually occurring as multiple lesions on the chest of children and young adults. Histology shows vellus hairs emerging from the cyst wall, and the condition is a developmental abnormality of vellus hair follicles. Spontaneous resolution may occur after a few years.

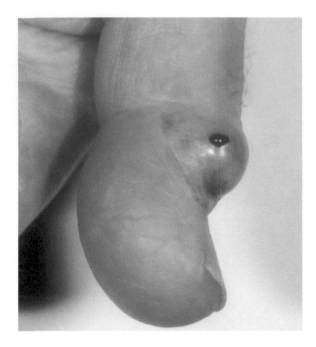

Figure 3.17 Mucoid (myxoid) cyst, showing a fluctuant lesion proximal to the thumb nail. Pricking the cyst with a sterile needle will produce the characteristic glistening viscous contents. Nail dystrophy is common if the cyst is adjacent to the nail fold.

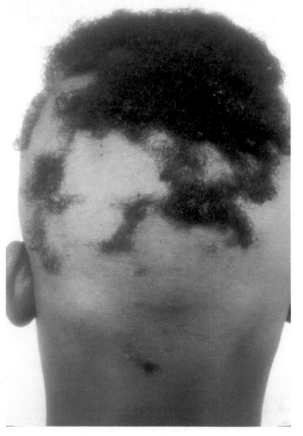

Figure 3.18 Alopecia areata, showing smooth, completely bald, non-scarred areas of skin on the scalp. These circular or oval patches of hair loss usually occur rapidly and the so-called 'exclamation mark' hairs may be apparent. It can be difficult to distinguish diffuse alopecia areata from other forms of diffuse hair loss, including iron deficiency or thyroid dysfunction. Complete loss of scalp hair is referred to as alopecia totalis and loss of all of the body hair, as alopecia universalis.

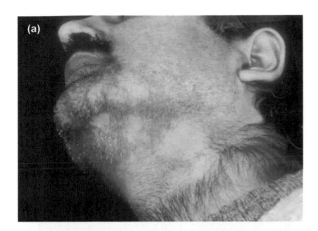

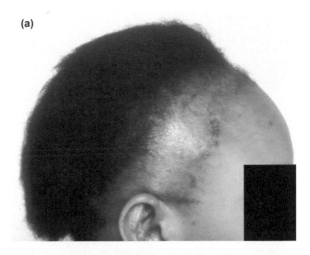

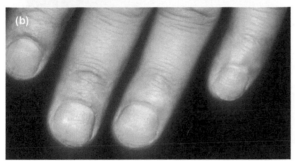

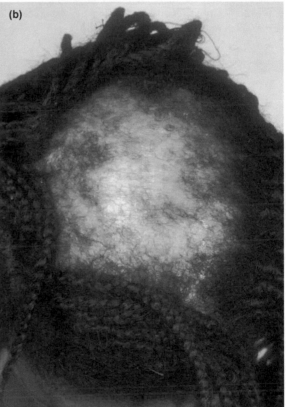

Figure 3.19a and b Alopecia areata, showing loss of hair from the beard area (3.19a) and nail dystrophy (3.19b). Alopecia areata is commonly familial and may be associated with a personal and/or family history of other autoimmune diseases such as vitiligo, pernicious anaemia, thyroiditis, and diabetes mellitus. Spontaneous regrowth of hair usually occurs over 18 months or so but poor prognostic indicators include nail dystrophy, loss of eyebrows and eyelashes, occipital involvement, and associated atopic dermatitis.

Figure 3.20a and b Traction alopecia results from constant traction on the hair (3.20a). It is less common in white people than in the past due to changing hair styles but is often seen in black women who brade their hair (3.20b), resulting from traction and sometimes the use of hot combs (hot comb alopecia). This is also referred to as central centrifugal alopecia.

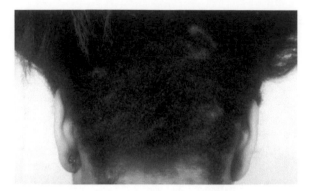

Figure 3.21 Trichotillomania, showing an extensive area of broken hairs on the occipital region of the scalp as a result of pulling, twisting, and/or rubbing the hair. Mild trichotillomania is quite common in children but there are sometimes serious underlying psychological problems which may persist into adulthood.

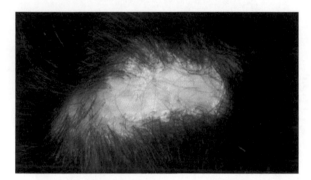

Figure 3.22 Folliculitis decalvans, showing a scarred linear area on the scalp vertex.

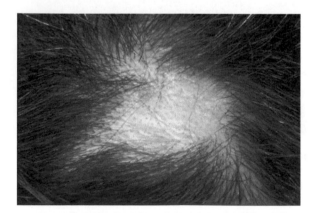

Figure 3.23 Alopecia neoplastica, showing sclerotic plaques on the scalp of a woman with carcinoma of the breast. This is a rare example of metastatic disease, nodular scalp deposits being more common.

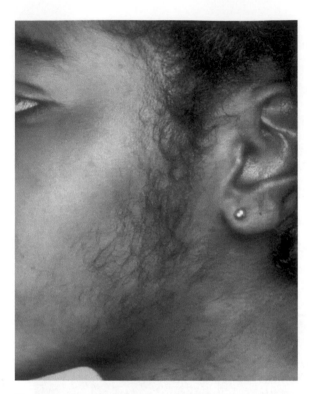

Figure 3.24 Hirsutism, in which there is excessive growth of terminal hair in the male distribution, is relatively common. Small amounts of excessive hair, particularly on the face, can cause great emotional upset but detailed endocrine investigations are usually not indicated unless extensive hirsutism is accompanied by abnormalities of the menstrual cycle.

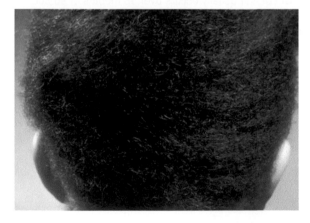

Figure 3.25 Pili torti, showing kinking of the hair in a white child. Each affected hair is flattened and irregularly twisted 180° on its own axis. This autosomal dominant disorder may occur alone or may be associated with keratosis pilaris, ichthyosis, dental and ocular abnormalities, and nerve deafness.

CHAPTER 4

Disorders of the dermal–epidermal interface and the dermis

LICHEN PLANUS
PITYRIASIS ROSEA

Disorders of the interface between the dermis and epidermis include the papulosquamous diseases, lichen planus, lichen nitidus, pityriasis rosea, chronic superficial scaly dermatitis, 'parapsoriasis' (Chapter 6), pityriasis lichenoides, seborrhoeic dermatitis (Chapter 2), and granuloma annulare (Chapter 6).

LICHEN PLANUS

Lichen planus is a well-defined skin disease in which the aetiology is obscure, although it is probably a tissue reaction to an unknown antigen, possibly a virus and occasionally a drug. In white skin, extremely itchy red or violaceous, flat-topped papules usually appear on the flexor aspects of the wrists, the forearms, and legs. With time, the violaceous colour is more obvious and a fine white epidermal network is seen on the surface of the lesions, the so-called Wickham's striae.

In black skin the papules are a deeper violaceous colour but the characteristic distribution of the lesions is often helpful, as is the presence of white lacey lesions on the buccal mucosa or lesions on the genitalia. The site of pathology is predominantly in the basal layer of the epidermis and upper (papillary) dermis. Disruption of melanocytes by the inflammatory process often leads to marked persistent hyperpigmentation in deeply pigmented skin (Chapter 1).

CHRONIC SUPERFICIAL SCALY DERMATITIS
PITYRIASIS LICHENOIDES

Lichen planus can cause scarring alopecia and severe nail dystrophy, and less common clinical variants include **annular lichen planus**, **hypertrophic lichen planus**, and **lichen planopilaris**.

> **Therapeutic suggestions**
> Topical corticosteroids
> Intralesional corticosteroids
>
> **Second-line treatment**
> Oral corticosteroids
> Oral retinoids

In **bullous lichen planus** the blisters are associated with lichen planus lesions, whereas in the rather rare disease **lichen planus pemphigoides** the blisters are usually also on normal-appearing skin.

Drugs known to cause **lichen planus-like (lichenoid) eruptions** include gold (sodium aurothiomalate), penicillamine, and mepacrine.

Lichen planus pigmentosus is a pigmentary disorder, recognized in patients of Asian Indian or Middle Eastern origin, in the presence or absence of lichen planus. The macular hyperpigmentation usually involves the face, neck, and upper limbs, but it may be more widespread (Chapter 1, Figure 1.7). There may be a slate grey or brownish-black appearance and the disorder can persist for 2 months to many years. Erythema dyschromicum perstans (ashy dermatosis), as described in South America, may be a macular variant of lichen planus pigmentosus (Chapter 10).

Lichen nitidus is uncommon and may or not be a variant of lichen planus. There are multiple asymptomatic tiny (pinhead sized) papules, each with a flat, shiny surface. In white skin the papules are 'skin coloured' but in black patients the shiny lesions are more noticeable, sometimes having a grey appearance.

> **Therapeutic suggestions**
> Topical corticosteroids

PITYRIASIS ROSEA

Pityriasis rosea is quite common in children and young adults and seems likely to be of viral origin, resolving spontaneously in about 6 weeks. Typically an individual red scaly patch on the trunk (the herald patch) is followed 2 or more days later by the development of erythematous oval scaly lesions on the trunk, upper arms, and thighs. The lesions on the trunk follow the line of the ribs, producing a 'Christmas tree' pattern. In black patients close inspection can sometimes reveal erythema in addition to post-inflammatory hyperpigmentation and, in the absence of erythema, one can usually appreciate scaling at the periphery of the lesions and the characteristic distribution of the eruption.

> **Therapeutic suggestions**
> Emollients
> Topical corticosteroids

CHRONIC SUPERFICIAL SCALY DERMATITIS

Chronic superficial scaly dermatitis (persistent superficial dermatitis, digitate dermatosis) is an uncommon disorder, in some ways resembling the eruption of the early stages of mycosis fungoides, but running a benign course, often for many years. There are usually multiple, superficial, slightly scaly plaques on the trunk and limbs, sometimes arranged in a digitate pattern. Histologically there is epidermal spongiosis, mild dermal oedema, and a sparse inflammatory cell (lymphocytic) infiltrate. Parapsoriasis is a confusing term which is probably best avoided (Chapter 6).

PITYRIASIS LICHENOIDES

Pityriasis lichenoides is probably a disease spectrum, comprising a more severe self-limited form, pityriasis lichenoides et varioliformis acuta, and a less severe persistent form, pityriasis lichenoides chronica.

Pityriasis lichenoides acuta is commoner in young people. The initial lesion is an oedematous pink papule, followed by a vesicle, then haemorrhagic necrosis. Scarring is variable and depends on the depth of the necrosis. The lesions occur in crops, particularly on the trunk, thighs, and upper arms. Even the acute form may last for a few months.

In **pityriasis lichenoides chronica (PLC)**, small reddish-brown papules occur on the trunk and medial aspect of the arms, each lesion having a characteristically adherent scale. The eruption is often persistent and typically improves with sun exposure.

> **Therapeutic suggestions**
> UVB
> Oral tetracycline

FURTHER READING

Bolognia JL, Jorrizzo JL, Rapini RP, et al (eds). Dermatology. Philadelphia: Mosby, 2003.

Burns T, Breathnach S, Cox N, Griffiths C (eds). Rook's Textbook of Dermatology, 7th edn. Oxford: Blackwell Science, 2004.

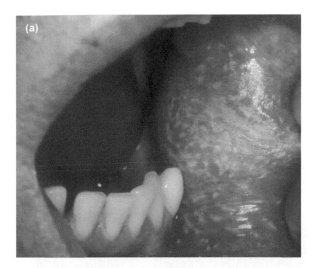 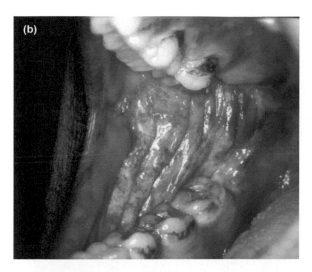

Figure 4.1a and b   Lichen planus, showing white papules on the buccal mucosa in a white person (4.1a) and papules accompanied by post-inflammatory hyperpigmentation in a black man (4.1b). Mucosal lesions are common and severe erosive changes are sometimes seen.

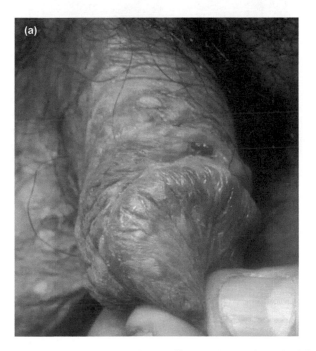 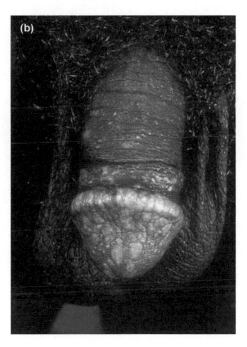

Figure 4.2a and b   Lichen planus affecting the penis, with violaceous papules on the corona of the glans (4.2a) and discrete papules on the glans and shaft of the penis (4.2b), the precise colour of the lesions depending partly on the background pigmentation.

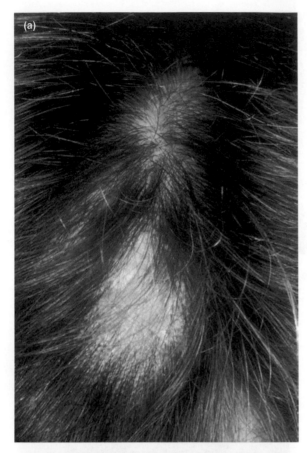

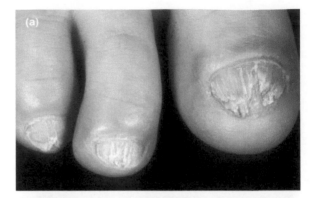

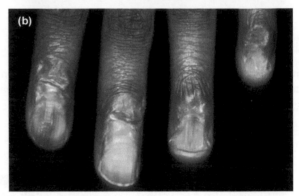

Figure 4.4a and b   Nail involvement in lichen planus. This is relatively uncommon, mild cases having pits and linear indentations. In severe examples there is marked linear dystrophy, as seen in the toenails (4.4a). The fingernails of a black person (4.4b), in which there is prominent inflammation of the nail fold region and pterigium formation (i.e. destruction of the nail which is replaced by scar tissue).

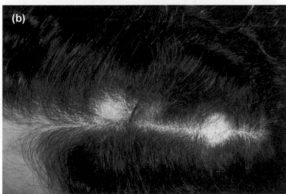

Figure 4.3a and b   Lichen planus, with scalp involvement leading to scarring alopecia: (4.3a) inflammation and some epidermal change; (4.3b) an active area of inflammation with two areas of scarring alopecia. The main differential diagnosis is discoid lupus erythematosus.

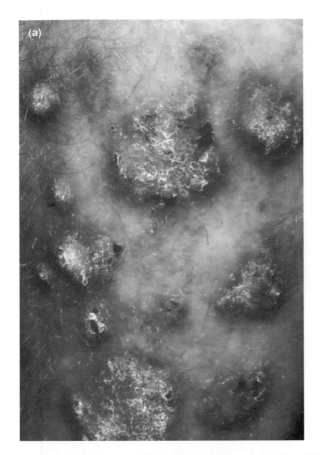
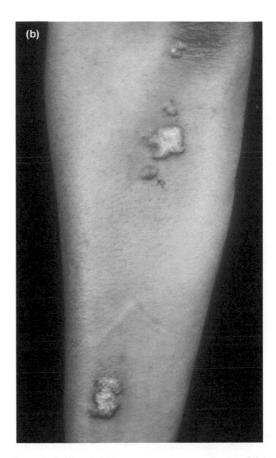

Figure 4.5a and b Hypertrophic lichen planus (4.5a) and lichen planus keloides (4.5b) are uncommon variants of lichen planus. Hypertrophic lichen planus on the limbs can be difficult to distinguish clinically from nodular prurigo.

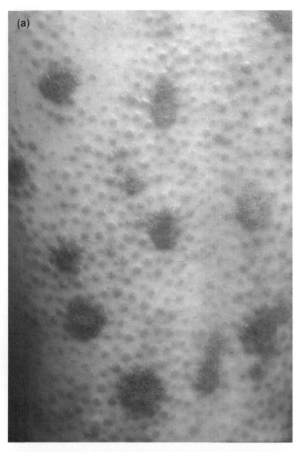

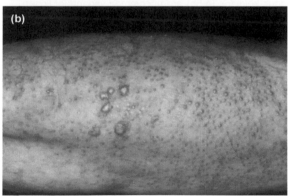

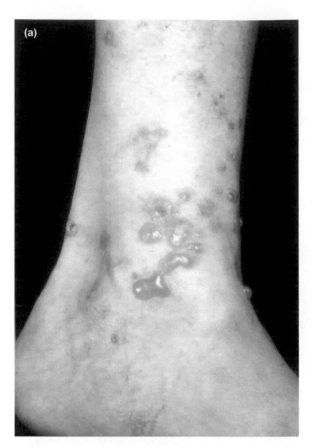

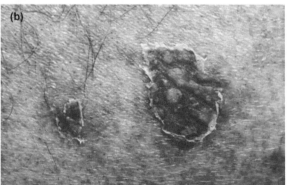

Figure 4.6a and b   Lichen planopilaris. Multiple papular lesions may be seen in the presence of other characteristic lichen planus lesions or sometimes as the only type of lesion. 4.6a shows violaceous papules and post-inflammatory hyperpigmentation on a limb, 4.6b showing typical lichen planus lesions and numerous follicular papules on the arm.

Figure 4.7a and b   Bullous lichen planus. (4.7a) Blisters associated with lichen planus lesions on the ankle. Lichen planus pemphigoides is a rare disease with immunofluorescent findings similar to bullous pemphigoid, in which the blisters may occur on either lesional or non-lesional skin. (4.7b) Erosions at the site of lichen planus lesion.

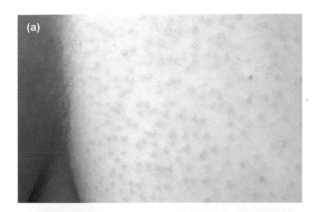

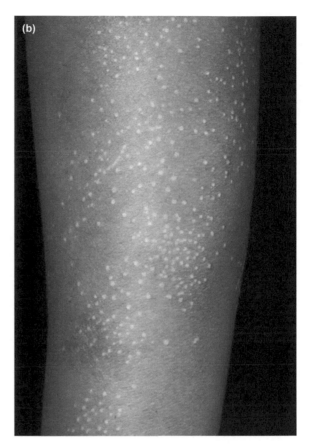

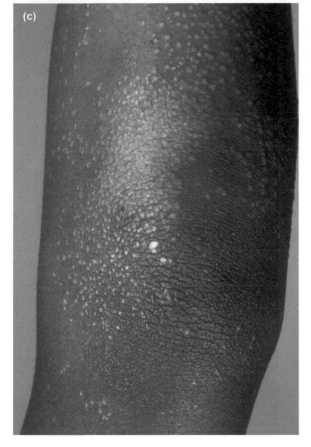

Figure 4.8a, b, and c Lichen nitidus, showing multiple tiny pink papules on the left upper arm (4.8a). In deeply pigmented skin, the papules are often a shiny grey colour (4.8b and c), sometimes accompanied by post-inflammatory hyperpigmentation (4.8c).

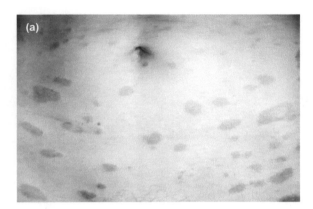

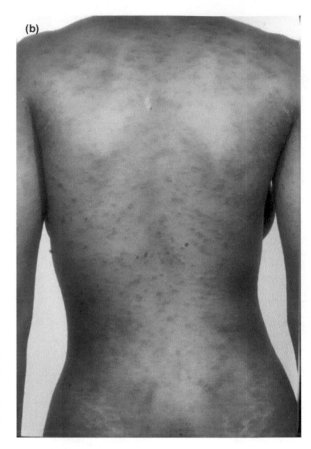

Figure 4.9a and b Pityriasis rosea, on the abdomen (4.9a), showing scaling macules. A solitary 'herald' patch may be seen on the day preceding the generalized eruption. Active inflammatory lesions can sometimes be seen in black patients, in whom one often sees post-inflammatory hyperpigmentation only (4.9b).

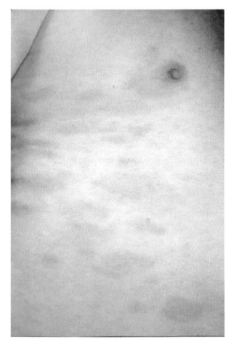

Figure 4.10 Chronic superficial scaly dermatitis (persistent superficial dermatitis), showing multiple superficial slightly scaly plaques on the side of the trunk, some of the lesions being arranged in a digitate pattern.

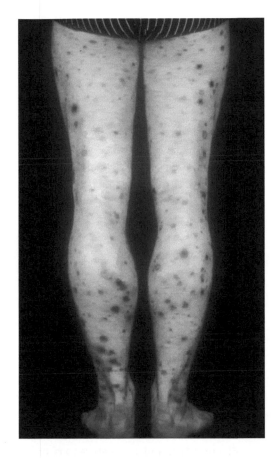

Figure 4.11   Pityriasis lichenoides acuta, showing prominent pink nodules and necrotic lesions on the legs.

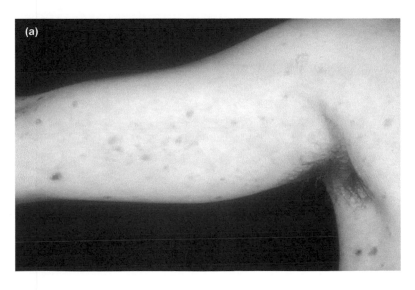

Figure 4.12a Pityriasis lichenoides chronica (PLC), with reddish scaly lesions on the medial aspects of the arms (4.12a). Close inspection of an individual lesion reveals a characteristic 'mica' scale.

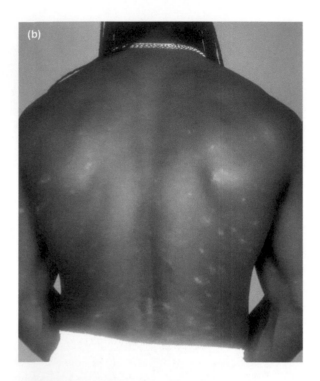

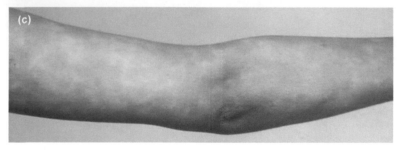

Figure 4.12b, and c Scaly lesions of PLC on the trunk of a man with deeply pigmented skin (4.12b). Post-inflammatory hypopigmented changes associated with PLC on the arm (4.12c).

CHAPTER 5

Disorders of epidermal and dermal–epidermal cohesion: blistering disorders

BULLOUS SKIN REACTIONS
IMMUNOBULLOUS DISEASES
MECHANOBULLOUS DISEASES

Broadly, the blistering disorders include those diseases in which blister (bulla or vesicle) formation can occur as a skin reaction to infective agents or drugs (erythema multiforme, toxic epidermal necrolysis), the immunobullous diseases (pemphigus, bullous pemphigoid, pemphigoid/herpes gestationis, dermatitis herpetiformis), and the mechanobullous diseases (epidermolysis bullosa), of which there are various types. Acquired epidermolysis bullosa, however, is an immunobullous disease. In children, the commonest causes of blistering are insect bite reactions and bullous impetigo.

BULLOUS SKIN REACTIONS

Erythema multiforme is a tissue reaction, sometimes to the herpes simplex virus or a drug (e.g. a sulphonamide), in which annular 'target' lesions develop, commonly on the hands and feet. Impending or frank blistering occurs at the dermal–epidermal junction and there is necrosis of the overlying epidermis; this is an example of an interface dermatitis.

> **Therapeutic suggestions**
> Aciclovir
>
> **Second-line treatment**
> Azathioprine
> Dapsone
> Thalidomide

Stevens–Johnson syndrome is an extreme form of erythema multiforme in which there is involvement of the oral, conjunctival, and genital mucosae, with systemic upset.

> **Therapeutic suggestions**
> Supportive measures
> Analgesia
>
> **Second-line treatment**
> Oral corticosteroids

In **toxic epidermal necrolysis (TEN)**, large areas of denuded skin occur, usually as a consequence of a drug allergy. There is some overlap clinically between

Stevens–Johnson syndrome and TEN. The distinction is important in that the use of systemic corticosteroids is controversial in established TEN because of concerns about sepsis. Larger prospective studies are required, but it seems that oral corticosteroids may help prevent the progression of TEN if given in the early stages of the disease.

Therapeutic suggestions
Supportive measures
Analgesia

Second-line treatment
Ciclosporin
Intravenous immune globulin

A skin biopsy can help distinguish TEN from **staphylococcal scalded skin syndrome** (SSSS), in which the epidermal necrosis is more superficial. These are diseases which require expert dermatological treatment and nursing care.

IMMUNOBULLOUS DISEASES

Pemphigus vulgaris is an uncommon, potentially fatal blistering disease which affects middle-aged or young adults. Oral erosions occur in about 50% of patients, often before the skin lesions. Superficial flaccid blisters or erosions are seen on the scalp, face, trunk, and flexures.

Therapeutic suggestions
Oral corticosteroids

Second-line treatment
Azathioprine
Mycophenolate mofetil
Intravenous immune globulin
Cyclophosphamide

Bullous pemphigoid is relatively common in the elderly, usually presenting with tense blisters on an erythematous or skin-coloured background, occurring on the trunk, limbs, and flexures. An uncomfortable pre-pemphigoid urticaria-like eruption may precede the blistering phase but oral ulceration is uncommon, occurring in only about 10%.

Therapeutic suggestions
Topical corticosteroids
Oral corticosteroids

Second-line treatment
Azathioprine
Dapsone
Tetracycline and nicotinamide
Methotrexate

Histopathological examination of a skin biopsy with direct immunofluorescence (IMF) of perilesional skin is necessary to confirm the precise diagnosis of an immunobullous disease. The commonest form of pemphigus is pemphigus vulgaris; rarer forms include **pemphigus foliaceus**, **pemphigus vegetans**, and **pemphigus erythematosus**. In pemphigus, the split is intraepidermal, whereas in bullous pemphigoid, **cicatricial pemphigoid** (the so-called benign mucosal pemphigoid), **linear IgA disease**, and pemphigoid gestationis (herpes gestationis), the level of blister formation is in the basement membrane, so that the bullae are subepidermal.

From a clinical point of view, the level of blister formation determines the likelihood of whether one sees erosions (as in pemphigus) or tense blisters (as in bullous pemphigoid). Oral ulceration is common in pemphigus vulgaris but unusual in bullous pemphigoid. However, mucosal involvement, with mouth and eye lesions, is frequently seen in cicatricial pemphigoid and linear IgA disease.

Table 5.1   Direct immunofluorescence in autoimmune blistering diseases

Disease	Pattern and type of immunoreactants
Pemphigus	Epidermal cell surface deposits of IgG and C3
Bullous pemphigoid	Linear homogeneous deposits of IgG (epidermal side on salt split skin) and C3 at the dermal–epidermal junction
Cicatricial pemphigoid	Linear homogeneous deposits of IgG and C3 at the dermal–epidermal junction
Linear IgA disease	Linear homogeneous deposits of IgA at the dermal–epidermal junction
Pemphigoid gestationis (herpes gestationis)	Linear homogeneous deposits of C3 at the dermal–epidermal junction
Dermatitis herpetiformis	Focal granular deposits of IgA in the dermal papillary tips
Epidermolysis bullosa acquisita	Linear homogeneous deposits of IgG (dermal side on salt split skin) and C3 at the dermal–epidermal junction

Direct IMF shows intercellular deposition of immunoglobulins (IgG, IgM) and complement components (C3) in the epidermis in pemphigus and basement membrane zone deposition in the various types of pemphigoid (Table 5.1). Indirect IMF to detect a circulating antibody is also usually performed, the antibody titre providing a useful indicator of disease activity in pemphigus vulgaris in particular.

Tzanck smears (see also Chapter 12) are performed less often than in the past, but may still be useful to rapidly confirm suspected pemphigus vulgaris. Bullae should be new and not infected with bacteria. The roof is removed and the floor scraped with a scalpel. In pemphigus, acantholytic cells can be observed, but further subclassification requires examination of histological specimens, with direct and indirect IMF.

In **dermatitis herpetiformis**, the blistering is subepidermal but vesicles are frequently not seen because of the intense itching and resultant excoriation. The scalp, buttocks, and elbows are characteristically involved and a skin biopsy is usually performed, direct IMF showing IgA in the papillary tips of the dermis (Table 5.1). The differential diagnosis includes eczema and scabies Dermatitis herpetiformis is associated with gluten-sensitive enteropathy, but this is often not clinically apparent.

Therapeutic suggestions
Dapsone
Gluten-free diet

Pemphigoid gestationis (herpes gestationis) is an extremely itchy disorder, occurring in the second or third trimester of pregnancy and recurring in subsequent pregnancies. Erythematous urticarial lesions, often accompanied by tense subepidermal blisters, usually begin on the abdomen but may affect any part of the body. The direct IMF findings are similar to those in bullous pemphigoid, with linear deposition of C3 along the basement membrane zone (Table 5.1).

Therapeutic suggestions
Topical corticosteroids
Oral antihistamines
Oral corticosteroids

Hailey–Hailey disease, also known as benign familial chronic pemphigus, is histologically similar to pemphigus vulgaris but with negative immunofluorescence findings. Characteristic erosions and erythema are seen in the axillae and groin region. A family history is common but not invariable. Friction and secondary bacterial infection play a role.

Therapeutic suggestions
Topical corticosteroids
Antibiotics

Aquired epidermolysis bullosa is the immunobullous type of epidermolysis bullosa (epidermolysis bullosa acquisita, EBA). EBA occurs in adult life, the clinical picture resembling porphyria but with positive direct immunofluorescent findings in the basement membrane zone. Using salt split skin IMF, antibodies bind to the dermal side (the floor) in EBA but mostly to the epidermal side (the roof) in bullous pemphigoid.

Therapeutic suggestions
Oral corticosteroids
Azathioprine
Dapsone

Second-line treatment
Colchicine
Intravenous immune globulin

MECHANOBULLOUS DISEASES

There are a number of other forms of epidermolysis bullosa (EB), which are rare inherited diseases, that may be scarring or non-scarring.

The characteristic feature of this group of diseases is the development of blistering on minimal trauma. **Epidermolysis bullosa simplex** is an autosomal dominant, usually mild, disorder, with a tendency to friction-induced blistering on the hands and feet (as seen when an infant crawls). The autosomal recessive **junctional epidermolysis bullosa** is rare, with large erosions occurring in the perioral and perianal regions at birth.

Epidermolysis bullosa dystrophica exists as an autosomal dominant and autosomal recessive form. In the autosomal dominant type, erosions heal with scarring and milia on the dorsum of the hands, elbows, and knees. The recessive type is a severe disease in which scarring may lead to fusion of the fingers and toes, with frequent mucosal (e.g. oesophageal) involvement. Recognition of the blistering diseases is not especially difficult in deeply pigmented skin, since one can generally see erosions or blistering. Pemphigus vulgaris has been reported to be a more severe disease in Indian patients. Even after early treatment, post-inflammatory hyperpigmentation can be particularly severe and persistent.

Specialist investigation of bullous diseases
Immunofluorescence:
   Direct IMF
   Indirect IMF
   Salt split skin IMF
Antigenic mapping
Prenatal diagnosis

FURTHER READING

Bolognia JL, Jorrizzo JL, Rapini RP, et al (eds). Dermatology. Philadelphia: Mosby, 2003.

Burns T, Breathnach S, Cox N, Griffiths C (eds). Rook's Textbook of Dermatology, 7th edn. Oxford: Blackwell Science, 2004.

Cerio R. Dermatopathology. In: Cerio R, Archer CB (eds). Clinical Investigation of Skin Disorders. London: Chapman and Hall Medical, 1998.

Dunnil MGS, Eady RAJ. Prenatal diagnosis of heritable skin diseases. In: Cerio R, Archer CB (eds). Clinical Investigation of Skin Disorders. London: Chapman and Hall Medical, 1998.

Lovell CR. General laboratory investigations. In: Cerio R, Archer CB (eds). Clinical Investigation of Skin Disorders. London: Chapman and Hall Medical, 1998.

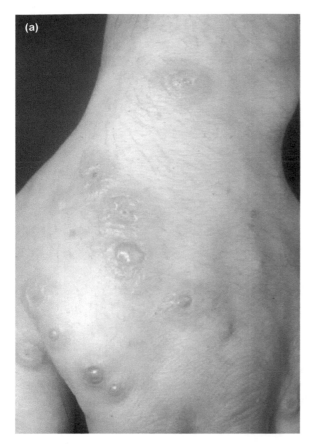

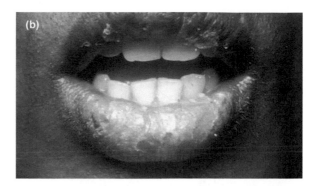

Figure 5.1a and b Erythema multiforme with erythematous blistered 'target' lesions on the dorsum of the hand (5.1a), and erythema and crusting of the lips in a black patient (5.1b). This clinical picture is commonly preceded by an infection with herpes simplex virus, and the characteristic skin lesions are not essential for the diagnosis.

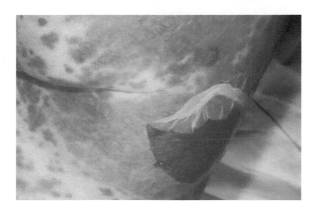

Figure 5.2 Toxic epidermal necrolysis, showing a sheet of denuded skin on the trunk of a woman in whom the initial red target-like lesions resembled Stevens–Johnson syndrome.

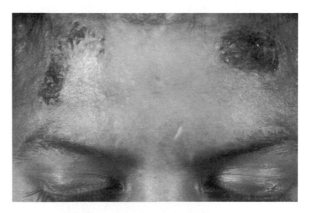

Figure 5.3 Pemphigus vulgaris, showing crusted erosions on the forehead of a man of Indian origin.

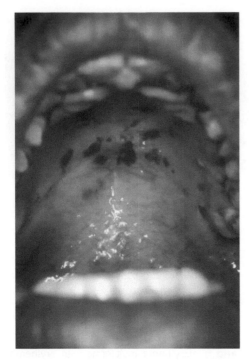

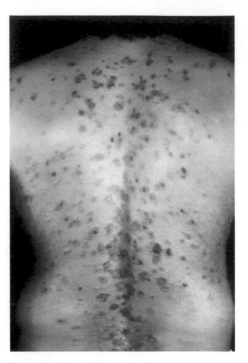

Figure 5.4 Oral ulceration is common in pemphigus vulgaris, as shown on the palate, and often precedes the development of skin lesions, which can occur insidiously.

Figure 5.5 Pemphigus foliaceus, with superficial erosions on the back of a man with deeply pigmented skin. This distribution is characteristic of pemphigus foliaceus and the split, confirmed by direct immunofluorescence, is in the upper part of the epidermis.

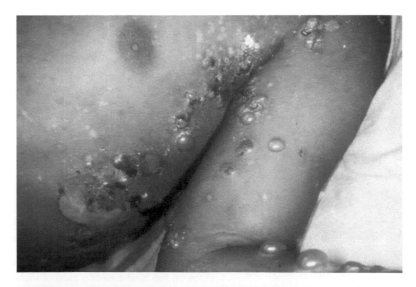

Figure 5.6 Bullous pemphigoid, with tense subepidermal blisters and erosions in deeply pigmented skin. Pemphigoid usually affects the elderly and the formation of blisters may be preceded by a prolonged prodromal erythematous eruption.

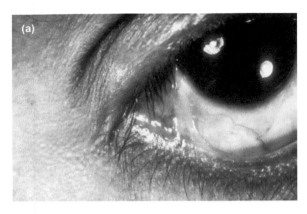

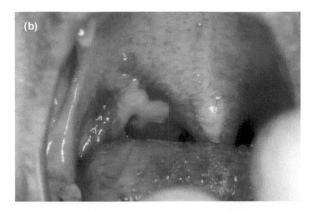

Figure 5.7a and b   Cicatricial pemphigoid, showing erosion and scarring of the conjunctiva (5.7a) and ulceration of the soft palate (5.7b).

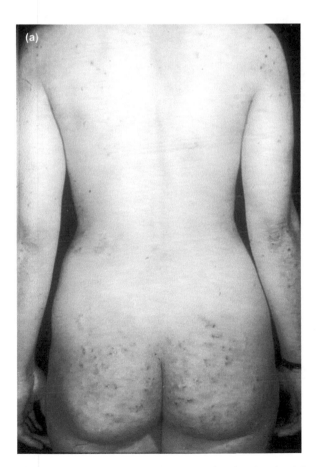

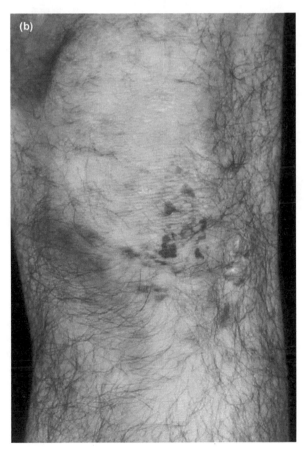

Figure 5.8a and b   Dermatitis herpetiformis, showing intensely itchy, excoriated lesions on the buttocks, elbows (5.8a), and knees (5.8b). The scalp and lower back are commonly involved and one frequently sees excoriations rather than vesicles.

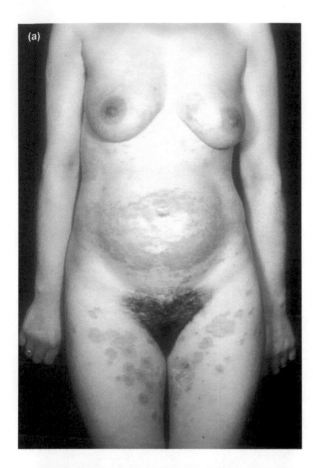

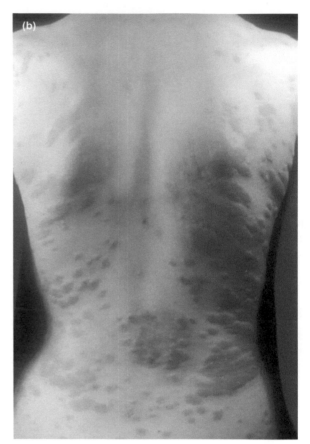

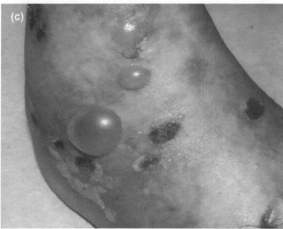

Figure 5.9 a, b, and c   Pemphigoid gestationis (herpes gestationis), showing erythematous urticarial lesions on the abdomen and thighs in the latter part of pregnancy (5.9a). Itchy urticarial areas are also prominent on the back (5.9b) and tense blisters, reflecting the subepidermal split, are a usual feature, as seen on the arm (5.9c).

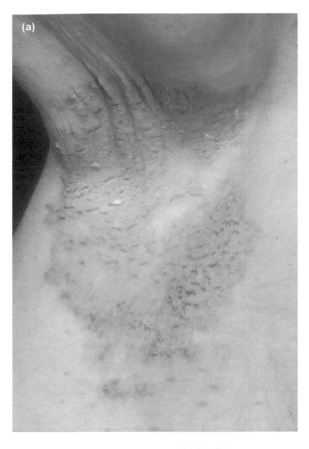

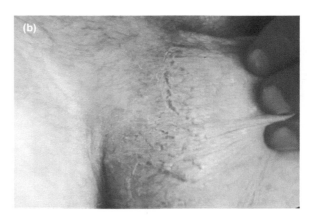

Figure 5.10a and b Benign familial chronic pemphigus (Hailey–Hailey disease) is histologically similar to pemphigus vulgaris but with negative immunofluoresence findings. Characteristic erosions and erythema are seen in the axilla (5.10a) and groin (5.10b). A family history is common but not invariable. Friction and secondary bacterial infection play a role.

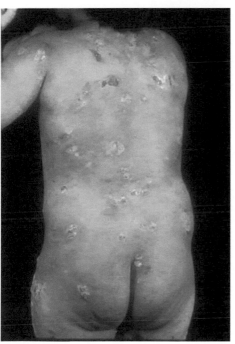

Figure 5.11 Epidermolysis bullosa simplex, showing thin-roofed blisters, erosions, and hyperkeratosis on the trunk and buttocks in a child with deeply pigmented skin. Blisters initially occur during infancy at sites of friction when the baby begins to crawl. Healing occurs without scarring but there may be some hyperpigmentation.

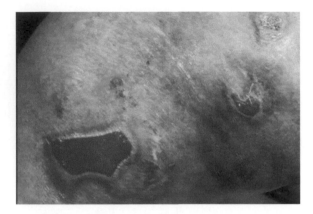

Figure 5.12 Epidermolysis bullosa dystrophica, showing deep erosions with scar formation in the pelvic region. This is the autosomal dominant type in which milia are often seen within the scars.

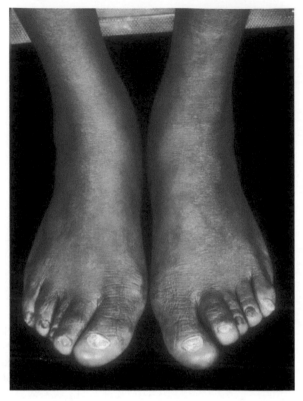

Figure 5.13 Epidermolysis bullosa, showing toe nail dystrophy in a young woman with deeply pigmented skin.

CHAPTER 6

Disorders of the dermis

BENIGN DERMAL DISORDERS
MALIGNANT DERMAL DISORDERS
Cutaneous T-cell lymphomas

Other malignant dermal diseases
CONNECTIVE TISSUE DISEASES
OTHER DERMAL ABNORMALITIES

Diseases solely or predominantly affecting the dermis include tumours derived from the cells of the dermis, various connective tissue diseases, and many of the cutaneous manifestations of systemic diseases (Chapter 8). Tumours involving the dermis may be benign or malignant, and sometimes provide the most obvious clinical features of inherited diseases, such as neurofibromatosis and tuberous sclerosis.

The diagnosis of dermal disorders in deeply pigmented skin does not usually present particular difficulties, since the level of pathology in the skin can often be established by palpation. However, difficulty in perceiving colour changes in black skin may pose diagnostic problems. For example, the purplish hue of vascular lesions is not seen in deeply pigmented skin and T-cell lymphoma is likely to present with persistent hyperpigmented or hypopigmented plaques or tumours rather than with erythematous plaques.

BENIGN DERMAL DISORDERS

Keloids are benign firm tumours usually resulting from an excessive connective tissue response to trauma, although they do sometimes occur spontaneously. Black patients are more likely to develop keloids than white patients and common sites include the chest, the upper back, the neck, and abdomen. Keloids may result from the trauma of ear piercing, surgery, burns, acne vulgaris (see Chapter 3), and

tattoos. It can be difficult to distinguish a keloid from a **hypertrophic scar**, the latter being confined to the area of trauma and tending to regress after 1–2 years. Both may be asymptomatic, painful or itchy, and can cause great cosmetic disability.

The treatment of keloids is aimed at softening and flattening the lesions and it is important for the patient's expectations to be realistic. Surgical excision may lead to a larger keloid and is ill-advised. The exception to this rule is in the management of earlobe keloids, which may not recur using appropriate compression following surgical excision. Intralesional corticosteroids and silicon gel are often used together routinely, with improvement of the keloids over a few months. Other treatments that have been tried with limited success include cryotherapy, laser therapy, excision followed by radiotherapy, and excision within the confines of the border of the keloid.

Therapeutic suggestions
Intralesional corticosteroids
Silicon gel

Second-line treatment
Cryotherapy
Laser therapy
Excision and radiotherapy

As discussed in Chapter 3, acne keloidalis nuchae can be very difficult to treat, but promising results have been reported following excision down to the fascia or deep subcutaneous tissue and healing by secondary intention.

Dermatofibromas (histiocytomas) are common, particularly on the legs, either occurring as a single lesion or a few lesions. **Leiomyomas** may be multiple or solitary, the complaint of pain often providing a clue to the diagnosis. **Juvenile xanthogranuloma** can occur as single or multiple lesions, each having a yellowish hue. In **neurofibromatosis** and **tuberous sclerosis** the distribution of the lesions is an important diagnostic aid.

Benign vascular lesions include **infantile haemangiomas**, which are benign developmental vascular tumours that appear during the first few months of life, and which characteristically have an initial proliferation and a later involutional phase. These are usually protuberant lesions and are sometimes referred to as capillary haemangiomas or strawberry naevi. Most but not all of them will resolve in the first 5 years.

A **port-wine stain** is a vascular malformation of developmental origin characterized pathologically by ectasia of superficial dermal capillaries and clinically by persistent macular erythema. Port-wine stains are not 'capillary haemangiomas' (a term used in older texts). On the face these disfiguring flat lesions may cause great psychological upset and they may be treated successfully with lasers, predominantly the pulsed dye laser.

This group of lesions also includes **spider naevi, arborizing telangiectasia, hereditary telangiectasia** (Osler–Rendu–Weber disease), **venous lakes, cherry angiomas** (Campbell de Morgan spots), which are common enough to be considered normal, **angiokeratomas** (seen in Anderson–Fabry disease), and **pyogenic granuloma.** Uncommon vascular lesions are **glomus tumours** (solitary or multiple), various forms of **poikiloderma, lymphoedema** and the uncommon, predominantly lymphatic vessel-derived entity, **lymphangioma circumscriptum.**

Jessner's benign lymphocytic infiltrate occurs as erythematous, raised, circular lesions on the face and upper trunk, usually in young adults. It runs a relapsing course and the main differential diagnosis is cutaneous discoid lupus erythematosus.

Ainhum is most common in Africans but also occurs in black Americans and other races. Patients usually present in adulthood (30–50 years old) with a painful fissure of the fifth toe, leading to clawing, and, eventually, once the constricting band encircles the digit, progressing to spontaneous amputation. Rest pain, cyanosis, and a cold distal digit suggest an ischaemic aetiology and, using arteriography, attenuation of the posterior tibial artery and absence of the plantar arch and its branches have been demonstrated. Mechanical and genetic factors may also be important. **Pseudo-ainhum** is a term used to describe other constricting bands, either congenital or acquired as a result of disease processes such as leprosy, scleroderma, neuropathy, trauma, or cold injury.

MALIGNANT DERMAL DISORDERS

Cutaneous T-cell lymphomas

Mycosis fungoides (MF), a form of primary cutaneous T-cell lymphoma (CTCL), is the most common dermal infiltrative malignancy. MF may occur in the form of slowly progressing plaques on the skin (early MF) or as an aggressive disease, sometimes presenting with obvious tumours. In plaque stage MF there is usually some clinical and histological evidence of epidermal involvement. Some patients with early MF do not progress further, whereas in others there is progression from small plaques to large plaques, to nodules, and later to ulcerated tumours and disseminated disease. Cutaneous T-cell lymphoma should be distinguished from lymphomatoid papulosis which runs a benign course, despite there being a clonal proliferation of T cells.

Follicular mucinosis may either be part associated with cutaneous T-cell lymphoma or a benign isolated finding. The clinical features of these two forms of follicular mucinosis are identical, with follicular papules and plaques, often associated with severe pruritus. There is a predeliction for the face and scalp, but the trunk and limbs may be affected.

The term **poikiloderma** describes the collective skin changes of telangiectasia, atrophy, and alternating areas of increased and decreased pigmentation, sometimes with scaling. In addition to being a feature of CTCL, it is seen in lupus erythematosus, dermatomyositis, drug eruptions, and in a number of congenital diseases.

Investigation of MF

Skin biopsy/biopsies:
  Routine histology
  Immunocytochemistry
  Molecular studies
Peripheral blood
  Routine haematology
  Biochemistry
  Serum lactate dehydrogenase (LDH)
  Sézary cells
  Lymphocyte subsets, CD4:CD8 ratio
  HTLV-1 serology
  TCR gene analysis of mononuclear cells*
Chest X-ray

Beyond stages IA and IB

Staging CT scans of the chest, abdomen, and pelvis

Advanced disease

Bone marrow aspirate and trephine biopsies

*These tests may be necessary to distinguish patients with acute T-cell leukaemia-lymphoma (ATLL) and those patients with peripheral blood T-cell clones who may have a poor prognosis.

Therapeutic suggestions

Topical corticosteroids
Emollients
PUVA
Topical nitrogen mustard

Second-line treatment

Local radiotherapy
Interferon-alpha-2a
Oral methotrexate
Oral or topical bexarotene
Total skin electron beam therapy

Parapsoriasis is a confusing term that is probably best avoided (Chapter 4). Parapsoriasis is sometimes divided into small-plaque parapsoriasis, which is considered to be the same as chronic superficial scaly dermatitis (CSSD), and large-plaque parapsoriasis, which may go on to develop into MF in about 10% of cases. In large-plaque parapsoriasis, patients present with persistent large yellow-orange atrophic patches and thin plaques on the trunk and limbs. Involvement of covered skin on the buttocks and breasts may suggest MF.

Sézary syndrome is a systemic form of CTCL in which there is erythroderma, lymphadenopathy, and >5% atypical mononuclear cells (Sézary cells) in the peripheral blood. Patients usually also complain of severe skin irritation or itching.

Other malignant dermal diseases

Systemic involvement is common when a **B-cell lymphoma** presents in the skin and such patients should be thoroughly investigated. Specific lesions, usually small reddish nodules, are more common in **monocytic leukaemia** than in other forms. Non-specific skin reactions in the leukaemias include purpura, pigmentation, pruritus, alopecia, exfoliative dermatitis, and herpes zoster. This group also includes **Langerhans cell histiocytosis** and the locally malignant tumour **dermatofibrosarcoma protuberans**.

Kaposi's sarcoma (KS) (see also Chapter 12) is a tumour composed of proliferating vascular and/or lymphatic channels, now well known because of its occurrence in the context of acquired immunodeficiency syndrome (AIDS). However, KS was observed before the 1980s as an uncommon tumour affecting the lower legs of elderly Italian, East European, or Jewish men. It was also known to be relatively common in young African adults and children, the latter subtype showing marked lymphatic involvement.

There is good evidence that the herpes virus HHV8 is the cause of KS. In elderly European males, a number of large purple plaques, each with overlying hyperkeratosis, initially develop on the feet and lower legs. In this type of KS, the disease is slowly progressive with the formation of oedema. In the African variety, oedema is frequently a presenting feature and the disease tends to rapidly progress to involve the lymph nodes, mucosal surfaces, and internal organs, particularly the small intestine.

CONNECTIVE TISSUE DISEASES

Dermal connective tissue diseases (see also Chapter 8) include morphoea, lichen sclerosus, and myxoedema. **Ehlers–Danlos syndrome** and **pseudoxanthoma elasticum** are rare genetic diseases which affect the collagen and elastin, respectively.

Morphoea usually presents with a localized firm white patch of sclerotic skin, initially with an inflamed border. The lesions may be linear, particularly in children, and in adults one commonly sees several brown macules on the trunk and limbs. Uncommonly the process, although limited to the skin, may be generalized.

Lichen sclerosus (lichen sclerosus et atrophicus, LSA) is a disorder affecting the vulva or glans penis (balanitis xerotica obliterans, BXO) and/or the skin. In many cases there is no atrophy, so the term lichen sclerosus is preferred. It is sometimes associated with morphoea.

Therapeutic suggestions
Topical corticosteroids
Emollients

Second-line treatment
Topical tretinoin
Circumcision

OTHER DERMAL ABNORMALITIES

Mucin deposition in the dermis occurs in a number of diseases, the most well-known being **pretibial myxoedema.** Raised reddish plaques occur on the shins, on the ankles, and dorsa of the feet, particularly after treatment of thyrotoxicosis.

Therapeutic suggestions
Topical corticosteroids with polythene occlusion
Intralesional corticosteroids

Necrobiosis lipoidica also occurs on the shins and other annular dermal lesions include granuloma annulare and sarcoidosis (Chapter 8).

The dermis is also the predominant site of pathology in disorders of exogenous aetiology, including **solar elastosis, radiodermatitis, corticosteroid-induced atrophy,** and **striae.**

FURTHER READING

Bolognia JL, Jorrizzo JL, Rapini RP, et al (eds). Dermatology. Philadelphia: Mosby, 2003.

Burns T, Breathnach S, Cox N, Griffiths C (eds). Rook's Textbook of Dermatology, 7th edn. Oxford: Blackwell Science, 2004.

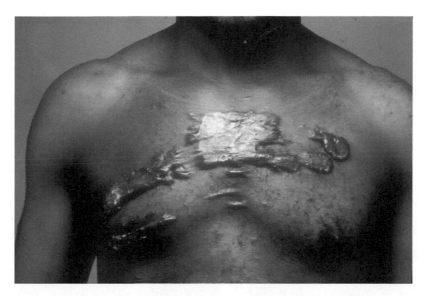

Figure 6.1   Keloids, showing disfiguring firm hyperpigmented lesions on the chest in a black man. Keloids can occur after trauma (e.g. surgery) or spontaneously, the scar tissue extending beyond the site of the original scar.

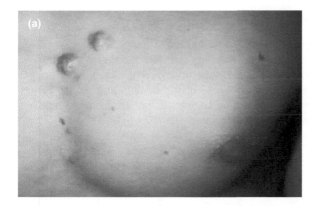

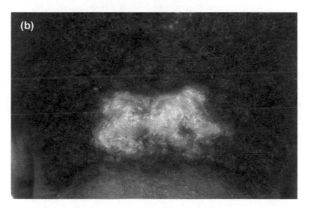

Figure 6.2a and b   Keloids associated with acne. 6.2a shows painful inflammatory lesions on the chest at the site of previous acne papules. Acne keloidalis nuchae (6.2b) is more common in black men, occurring on the nape of the neck above or below the hairline.

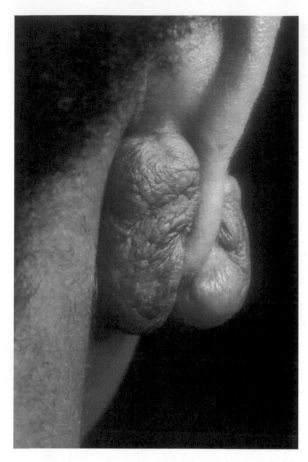

Figure 6.3   Keloids, following piercing of the earlobes. Keloid formation at this site does not necessarily imply that keloids will form at other sites after trauma. Surgical excision may be successful in this situation but is usually contraindicated at other sites.

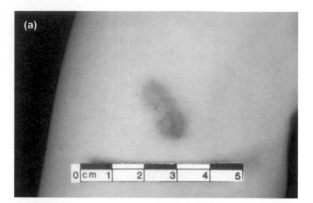

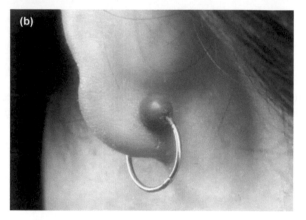

Figure 6.4a and b   (6.4a) Hypertrophic scar, showing a reddish sore inflammatory scar on the upper arm. Unlike with a keloid, the hypertrophic scar tissue does not extend beyond the site of the original scar. (6.4b) An earring granuloma, a complication of ear piercing, to be distinguished from a keloid.

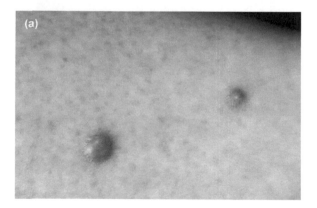

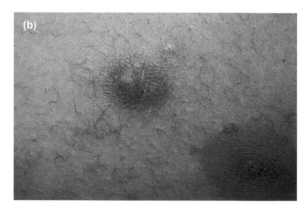

Figure 6.5a and b   Dermatofibroma (histiocytoma), showing two pink firm nodules on the lower leg in white skin (6.5a). Lesions are initially cellular and later become fibrotic, often with the development of brown pigmentation. In black skin dermatofibromas are firm hyperpigmented lesions, as seen on the chest near the areola of the breast in an African man (6.5b).

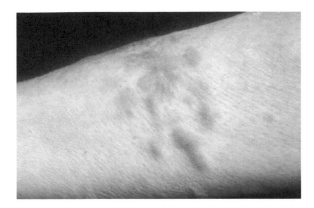

Figure 6.6 Leiomyoma, showing a group of painful pink nodules on the wrist of a white woman. The clue to diagnosis is the symptom of pain within the lesions, occurring either spontaneously or after exercise, minimal trauma, or exposure to cold, presumably related to contraction of the arector pilaris muscles.

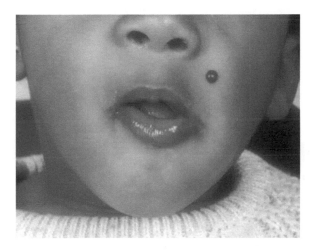

Figure 6.7 Juvenile xanthogranuloma, showing a solitary nodule on the cheek of a young boy. Characteristically a xanthogranuloma has a yellowish colour, masked by hyperpigmentation in this child with deeply pigmented skin.

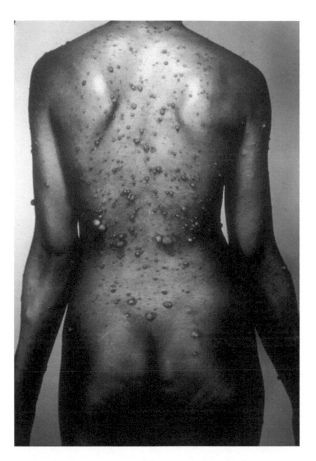

Figure 6.8 Type 1 neurofibromatosis, showing characteristic protuberant lesions on the trunk. In black skin the lesions are often hyperpigmented. Patients often have café au lait macules, axillary freckling, and a family history of neurofibromatosis.

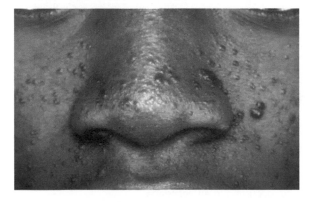

Figure 6.9 Tuberous sclerosis, showing numerous dark-coloured angiofibromas in the paranasal area. The facial lesions are not sebaceous adenomas, so that the term 'adenoma sebaceum' is a misnomer.

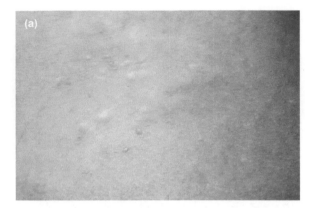

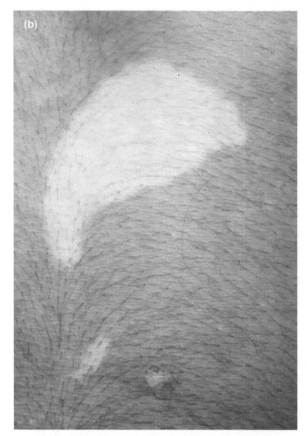

Figure 6.10a and b Tuberous sclerosis, showing a 'shagreen patch' on the lower back (6.10a) and the less specific hypopigmented 'ash leaf macule' on the back (6.10b). These are earlier features of the disease, sometimes noted after the child presents with a convulsion.

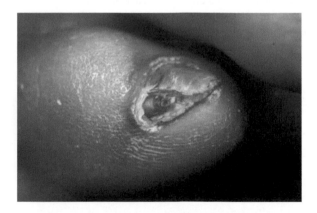

Figure 6.11 Tuberous sclerosis, showing a periungual fibroma on a toe. These can also affect the fingers and, as with angiofibromas, are relatively late features of the disease, occurring in adolescence.

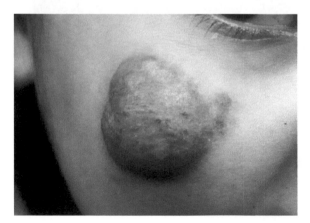

Figure 6.12 Strawberry naevus, a protuberant vascular malformation on the cheek of a child. Strawberry naevi usually develop in the first few days of life and tend to spontaneously resolve over the next 5 years.

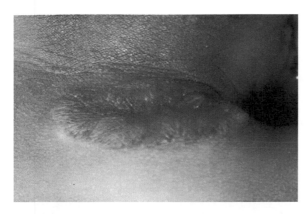

Figure 6.13 Strawberry naevus, with evidence of spontaneous resolution on the nape of the neck in a black child. Impairment of vision is an indication for early treatment with an appropriate laser.

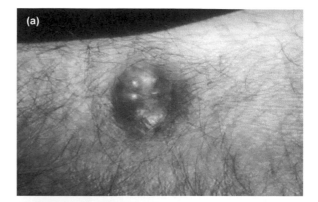

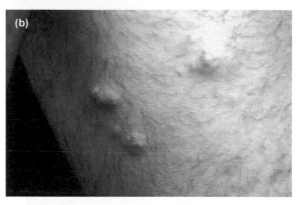

Figure 6.15a and b Glomus tumour, showing a solitary painful nodule on the arm (6.15a) and multiple soft vascular lesions on the upper arm in a man with deeply pigmented skin (6.15b). The tumours are usually painful and may be subungual.

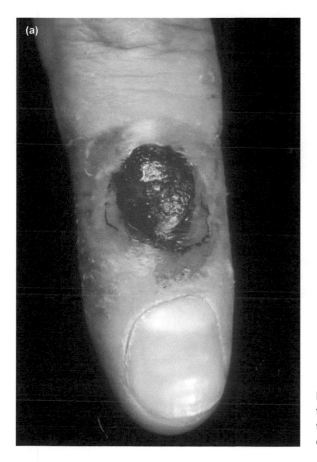

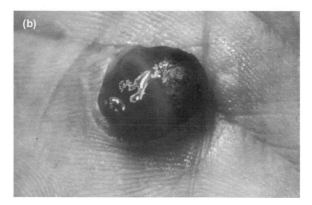

Figure 6.14a and b Pyogenic granuloma (granuloma telangiectaticum), shown on the finger (6.14a) and palm of the hand (6.14b). These protuberant vascular lesions develop rapidly and sometimes have a pus-covered surface.

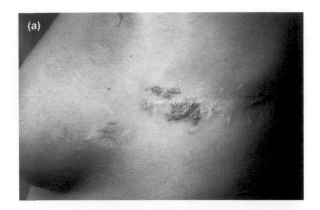

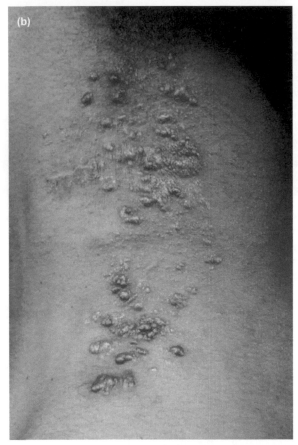

Figure 6.16a and b   Lymphangioma circumscriptum, with purplish hyperpigmented fluid-filled lesions on the trunk (6.16a) and neck (6.16b).

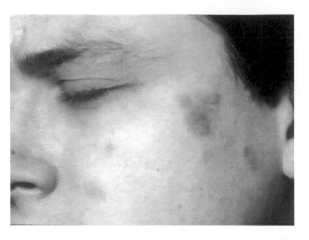

Figure 6.17   Jessner's benign lymphocytic infiltrate, showing red infiltated lesions on the face. Typically, lesions occur in relapsing fashion on the face and upper trunk of young adults. The main differential diagnosis is cutaneous lupus erythematosus.

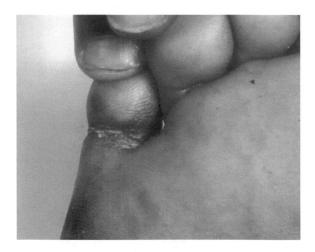

Figure 6.18   Ainhum, showing a painful constrictive fissure of the fifth toe in an African man. Spontaneous amputation eventually occurs.

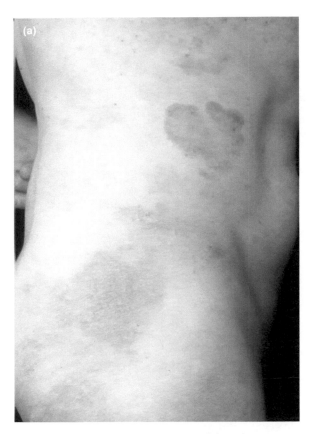
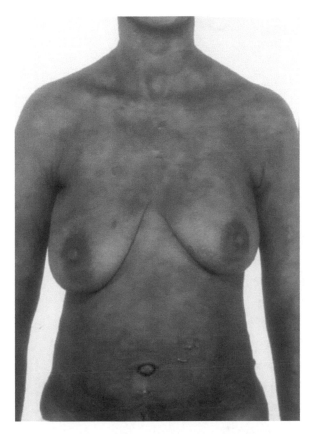

Figure 6.19a and b Mycosis fungoides (a form of cutaneous T-cell lymphoma), showing erythematous plaques on the trunk and pelvic region in a white man (6.19a) and hyperpigmented plaques on the arms and trunk of a black woman (6.19b). Histological confirmation of cutaneous T-cell lymphoma is essential.

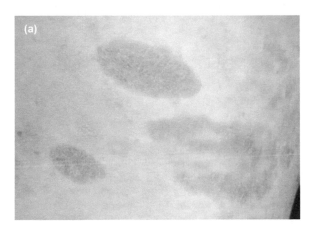
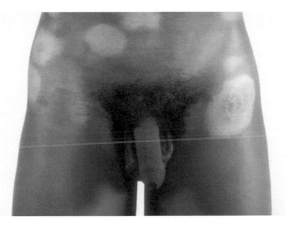

Figure 6.20a and b Mycosis fungoides, showing telangiectatic red plaques on the trunk (6.20a) and, in a black man, hypopigmented plaques on the abdomen and thighs (6.20b). This disease is commonly confined to the skin and only slowly progressive.

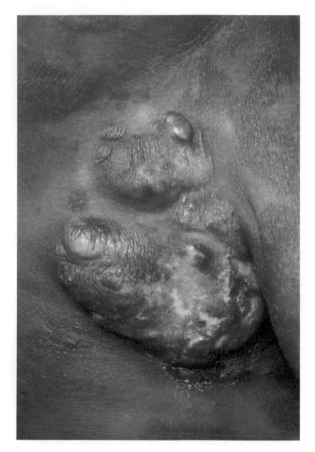

Figure 6.21 Mycosis fungoides, with tumour stage disease on the trunk. The clinical course of cutaneous T-cell lymphoma is variable. Patients who present with large exophytic tumours and should be investigated for systemic involvement.

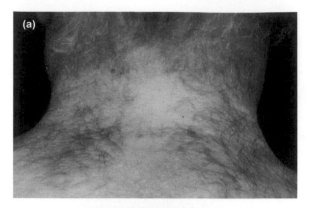

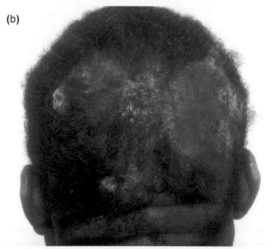

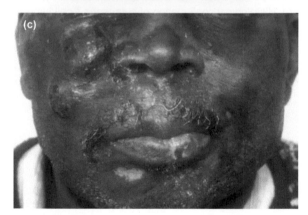

Figure 6.22a, b and c Follicular mucinosis, showing areas of hair loss on the nape of the neck and upper back (6.22a) and the scalp (6.22b). The erythema is not apparent in the black patient (6.22b). 6.22c shows extensive facial involvement in a man of Afro-Caribbean origin who had HTLV-1-associated T-cell lymphoma, subsequently reclassified as acute T-cell leukaemia-lymphoma (ATLL). Follicular mucinosis may also occur as a benign isolated finding.

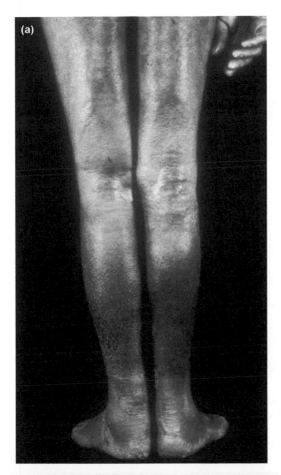

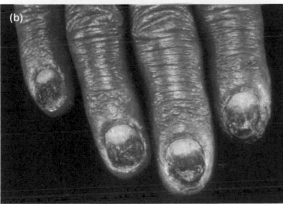

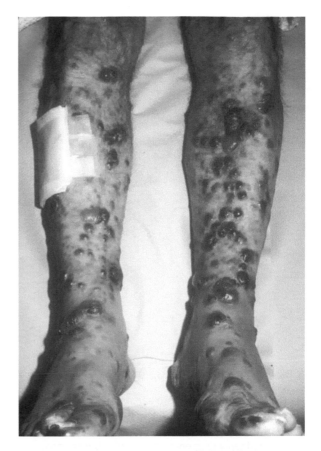

Figure 6.24 B-cell lymphoma. Bullous lesions may occur in association with the more usual nodules of B-cell lymphoma and systemic involvement at the time of cutaneous presentation is more common than with T-cell lymphoma.

Figure 6.23a and b Sézary syndrome, showing hyper-pigmentation on the legs (6.23a) and nail changes (6.23b) in a black man. The nail changes are not specific and may be seen in other forms of erythroderma. There is a spectrum of severity in Sézary syndrome and different subgroups may exist, some patients being extremely ill with intractable pruritus.

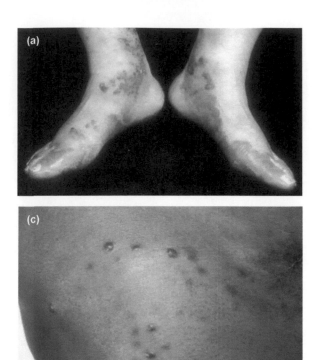

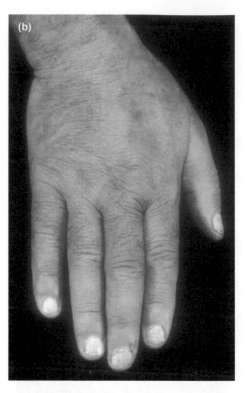

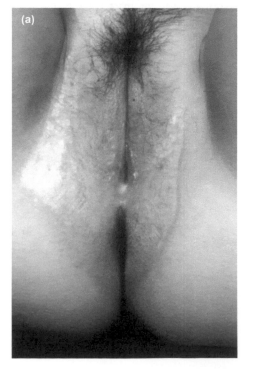

Figure 6.25a, b and c   Kaposi's sarcoma, showing purplish plaques on the ankles and feet (6.25a), with diffuse vascular lesions on the dorsum of the hand (6.25b). This chronic form of Kaposi's sarcoma occurs in the absence of HIV infection in elderly men of Jewish, Italian, or East European origin. 6.25c shows grouped hyperpigmented nodules on the trunk of a man with deeply pigmented skin, a distribution more characteristic of AIDS-associated Kaposi's sarcoma.

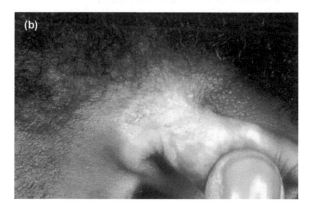

Figure 6.26a and b   Lichen sclerosus et atrophicus (LSA), showing white atrophic areas of skin in the perivulval and perianal region (6.26a) and above the ear (6.26b). Lesions are commonly extremely itchy. Other sites include the glans penis (balanitis xerotica obliterans) and the trunk. LSA and morphoea sometimes coexist.

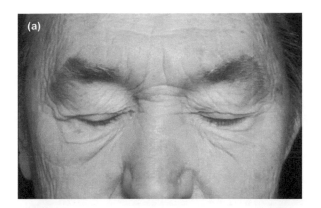

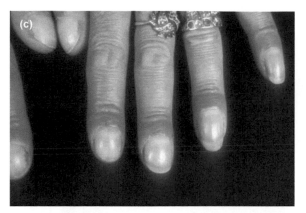

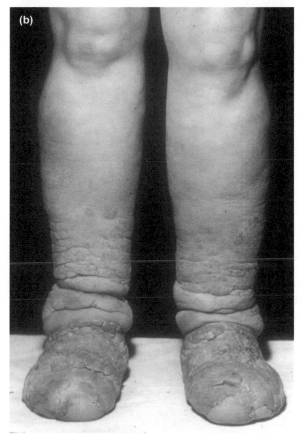

Figure 6.27a, b and c   Myxoedema, showing periocular mucinous infiltration and loss of the lateral eyebrows in a man with hypothyroidism (6.27a). 6.27b shows the late changes of severe pretibial myxoedema following treatment of thyrotoxicosis and 6.27c shows the features of thyroid acropatchy.

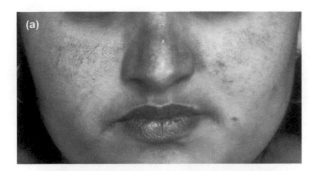

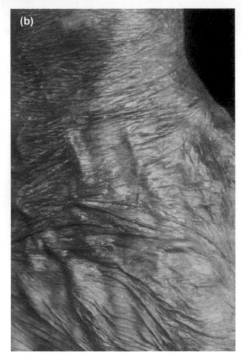

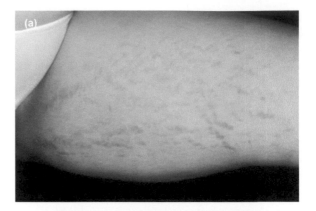

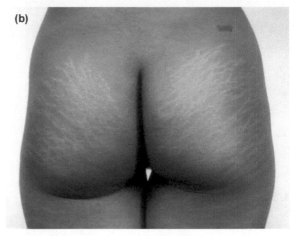

Figure 6.28a and b   Corticosteroid-induced atrophy of the skin on the face (6.28a) and on the dorsum of the hand (6.28b), following the prolonged application of fluorinated topical corticosteroids. Telangiectasia (6.28a) and larger blood vessels (6.28b) are readily visible. On the face there is often an associated acneiform perioral dermatitis.

Figure 6.29a and b   Striae, on the inner thighs of a young white woman after prolonged use of fluorinated topical corticosteroids (6.29a). 6.29b shows striae on the buttocks of a black woman. In white skin, striae are reddish-purple in colour whereas they are commonly hypopigmented in deeply pigmented skin. In the absence of topical corticosteroids, striae usually follow stretching of the skin, as occurs during pregnancy or after rapid growth in children.

CHAPTER 7

Disorders of the vasculature and subcutaneous disorders

SKIN ULCERATION
Leg ulcers and pressure sores
Pyoderma gangrenosum

VASCULITIS
SUBCUTANEOUS DISORDERS

SKIN ULCERATION

Leg ulcers and pressure sores

The majority of leg ulcers are **venous (gravitational) ulcers**, commonly occurring in women and often associated with previous thrombosis of the deep venous system. Ulceration frequently involves the medial malleolar region, and there is often purplish-brown discoloration and white fibrosis with purpura of the surrounding skin (atrophie blanche). Varicose eczema and varicose veins are commonly associated with venous ulcers.

Important aspects of treatment include elevation and adequate compression or elastic support, such as the 4-layer bandage system, once Doppler (ultrasound) studies have been performed to make sure the arterial supply is not significantly impaired. A number of dressings have been developed, the aim of which is to keep the ulcer moist and free from infection. In the absence of signs of infection, such as cellulitis, a wound swab from the ulcerated surface may be misleading.

> **Therapeutic suggestions**
> Compression for venous ulcers

> **Second-line treatment**
> Oral pentoxifylline
> Skin equivalent dressings

Arterial leg ulcers are usually painful, especially when the legs are elevated. The ulcers are often multiple and have a punched out appearance. In the elderly, it is often difficult to palpate peripheral pulses and assessment by Doppler studies is these days considered essential. This can directly affect the management of the patient with arterial ulceration, in which elevation and supportive bandaging would be inappropriate.

Leg ulcers are also associated with diabetes mellitus, rheumatoid arthritis, polyarteritis nodosa, haemolytic anaemia, acute cutaneous infections, and syphilis. Pyoderma gangrenosum may occur on the legs, when there may be a venous component to the overall process. In patients of African origin, there is an increased prevalence of **sickle cell disease**, which is associated with leg ulcers.

Pressure sores (decubitus ulcers) commonly occur over the sacrum but can also affect the legs and feet. Prevention by good nursing care is so important.

Pyoderma gangrenosum

Pyoderma gangrenosum (PG) is an uncommon non-infectious neutrophilic dermatosis commonly associated with underlying systemic disease. Several clinical variants of PG have been described, including ulcerative, pustular, bullous, and vegetative forms. An immune-mediated process is thought to play an important pathogenetic role, with about 50% of patients having an associated systemic disease. Common associations include inflammatory bowel diseases (ulcerative colitis and Crohn's disease), rheumatoid arthritis, haematological malignancies, and monoclonal gammopathies.

A characteristic presentation of PG begins with small tender papules or pustules that evolve into painful ulceration with typical undermined violaceous edges. Different skin sites may be involved, including peristomal skin. Healing usually occurs with an atrophic cribriform scar (i.e. having a number of small holes within it). Bullous PG is often associated with myeloproliferative disorders. Vegetative (superficial granulomatous) PG may have superficial and deep components and is not usually associated with any systemic disease.

The diagnosis of PG is made by recognizing the characteristic clinical features and by excluding other causes of ulceration. A biopsy across the edge of a lesion, depending on the type of PG, will show a neutrophilic infiltrate, but at best the histology is 'consistent with' as opposed to 'diagnostic of' PG.

Therapeutic suggestions
Topical tacrolimus
Topical corticosteroids
Minocycline
Oral corticosteroids

Second-line treatment
Ciclosporin
Infliximab

VASCULITIS

Vasculitis is a pathological process of inflammation and damage primarily involving the blood vessel walls, resulting in purpura, nodules, and sometimes ulceration. A number of clinical variants have been described; one subclassification is based on the predominant cell type involved – one may see a neutrophilic, lymphocytic, or granulomatous vasculitis.

The neutrophil-rich skin lesions of **polyarteritis nodosa** (PAN), **hypersensitivity (allergic) vasculitis**, and **Henoch-Schönlein purpura** (more commonly occuring in children) are usually part of a systemic disease, although cutaneous polyarteritis nodosa does occur. Once the diagnosis of leukocytoclastic vasculitis has been confirmed histologically, investigations are directed towards finding the cause and the degree of systemic involvement.

Investigation of vasculitis
Diagnosis
Skin biopsy (of an early lesion)

Cause
FBC and differential WCC
ESR or viscosity
ASO and anti-DNase B titres
Rheumatoid factor
Antinuclear antibodies
Complement C3 and C4
Hepatitis B and C serology
Antineutrophil cytoplasmic antibodies (ANCAs):
    perinuclear ANCA (pANCA)
    cytoplasmic ANCA (cANCA)
Plasma cryoglobulins*
α_1-Antitrypsin
Serum amylase and urine lipase

Systemic involvement
Urine for protein, red cells, and casts
Serum creatinine and urea
More specific tests of renal function
Blood cultures
Echocardiography

*To look for plasma cryoglobulins, a fasting blood sample should be allowed to clot at 37°C for 3–4 hours. The serum is then cooled at 4°C for several days.

Therapeutic suggestions
Observation
Withdrawal of the cause
Colchicine
Dapsone

Second-line treatment
Oral corticosteroids

Therapeutic suggestions
Non-steroidal anti-inflammatory drugs

Second-line treatment
Potassium iodide
Colchicine
Oral corticosteroids
Dapsone

A characteristic feature of hypersensitivity vasculitis is the occurrence of palpable purpura, in contrast to the reddish purpuric lesions of the various patterns of **capillaritis** (pigmented purpuric eruptions). **Erythema elevatum diutinum** is a rare form of vasculitis which presents with purplish plaques on the knees or dorsa of hands.

Erythema nodosum (a form of panniculitis), pityriasis lichenoides et varioliformis acuta, and pityriasis lichenoides chronica (Chapter 4), and **chilblains** are examples of a lymphocytic vasculitis. The granulomatous vasculitides such as **Wegener's granulomatosis** and **erythema induratum** (nodular vasculitis, Bazin's disease) are rare. Erythema induratum is associated with tuberculosis and is more common in UK patients of Indian Asian origin.

SUBCUTANEOUS DISORDERS

The various types of **panniculitis** are classified by histological pattern and by the presence or absence of vasculitis. Panniculitis has been classified as septal panniculitis, lobular panniculitis, mixed panniculitis, and panniculitis with vasculitis.

Erythema nodosum is an example of septal panniculitis in which the inflammatory changes also involve the overlying dermis. There are usually painful bruise-like lesions on the shins. Erythema nodosum may be provoked by a number of stimuli, including streptococcal infection, drugs (including oral contraceptives and sulphonamides), sarcoidosis, and tuberculosis. The patient may be unwell with fever and arthralgia, and the lesions usually resolve in a few weeks.

Relapsing febrile nodular panniculitis (Weber–Christian syndrome) and idiopathic nodular panniculitis are examples of lobular panniculitis. Subcutaneous panniculitis simulating Weber– Christian syndrome may be associated with α_1-antitrypsin deficiency. Lupus panniculitis, usually known as lupus profundus, is a form of mixed (septal and lobular) panniculitis. When carrying out a skin biopsy it is essential to include subcutaneous tissue, otherwise the pathology may be missed.

Lipomas are common benign subcutaneous tumours which may be multiple. Rare disorders of the subcutis include total and partial lipodystrophy (lipoatrophy). **Total lipodystrophy** may be congenital, acquired, and/or familial. There is loss of subcutaneous and visceral fat, hepatomegaly, increased bone growth, hyperlipaemia, and subsequently diabetes mellitus. Diabetes mellitus is also sometimes associated with **partial lipodystrophy**, which usually affects children or young adults.

Malignant atrophic papulosis (Degos' disease) is a rare infarctive abnormality of the vessels in the subcutaneous fat and internal organs. Death usually occurs within a few years from intestinal perforation or cerebral infarction.

FURTHER READING

Bolognia JL, Jorrizzo JL, Rapini RP, et al (eds). Dermatology. Philadelphia: Mosby, 2003.

Burns T, Breathnach S, Cox N, Griffiths C (eds). Rook's Textbook of Dermatology, 7th edn. Oxford: Blackwell Science, 2004.

Lovell CR. General laboratory investigations. In: Cerio R, Archer CB (eds). Clinical Investigation of Skin Disorders. London: Chapman and Hall Medical, 1998.

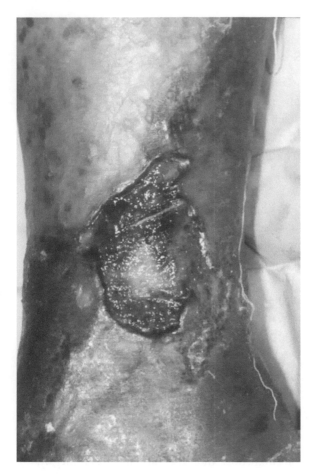

Figure 7.1 Chronic venous insufficiency, with a venous ulcer over the medial malleolus, a common site.

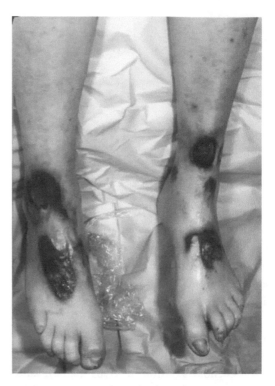

Figure 7.3 Diabetic leg ulceration, affecting the dorsa of the feet and anterior ankle region. The ulcers usually occur at sites of trauma, e.g. when a foot rubs on a shoe or a heel rests on the bed. Other pathogenic factors in diabetes mellitus include microvascular abnormalities, peripheral neuropathy, and impaired ability to deal with infection.

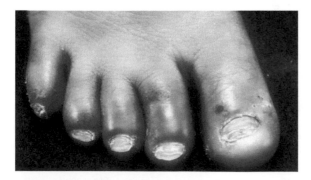

Figure 7.2 Arterial ischaemia. This may be acute (e.g. after an embolus) or chronic (e.g. atherosclerosis). This figure shows painful purplish discoloration of the toes. Frank ulceration of the distal extremity can occur.

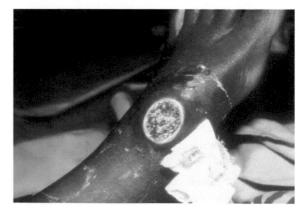

Figure 7.4 Tropical ulcer, occurring at the site of trauma on the dorsum of the foot. A number of factors may be involved in the aetiology and the spirochaete *Borrelia vincentii*, amongst other organisms, has been implicated. In a young black patient, leg ulceration should also alert the physician to the possibility of sickle-cell anaemia.

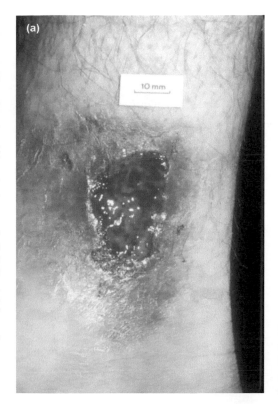

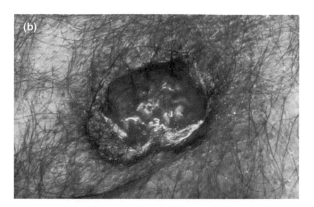

Figure 7.5a and b Pyoderma gangrenosum, showing ulceration with characteristically undermined edges. Pyoderma gangrenosum is associated with rheumatoid arthritis, Crohn's disease (as in 7.5a), ulcerative colitis, and other underlying diseases.

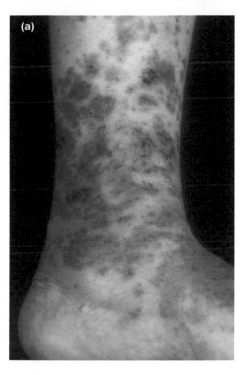

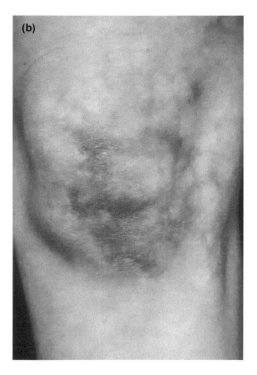

Figure 7.6a and b   Vasculitis, showing reddish palpable purpuric lesions and ulceration on the lower leg (7.6a). Vasculitis can be accompanied by a network of violaceous streaks, described as livedo reticularis (7.6b).

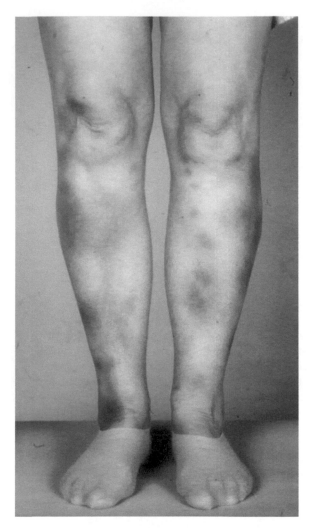

Figure 7.7 Erythema nodosum, with painful bruise-like lesions on the shins. This may be regarded as a lympho-cytic vasculitis or panniculitis, provoked by a number of stimuli, including streptococcal infection, drugs (e.g. sulphonamides), sarcoidosis, and tuberculosis. The patient may be unwell with fever and arthralgia and the lesions usually resolve in a few weeks.

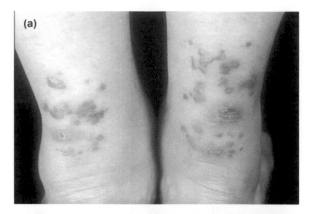

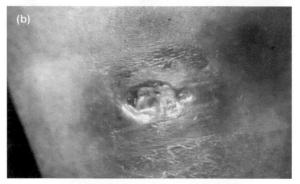

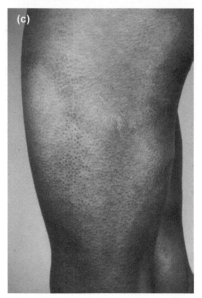

Figure 7.8a, b, and c Panniculitis, showing reddish nodules on the lower calves in a woman with Bazin's dis-ease (erythema induratum), a tuberculide (7.8a). 7.8b shows another example of a nodular form of vasculitis, with ulceration and surrounding hyperpigmentation. 7.8c shows a painful subcutaneous nodule on the posterior thigh of a black man with panniculitis and incidental keratosis pilaris (Chapter 2).

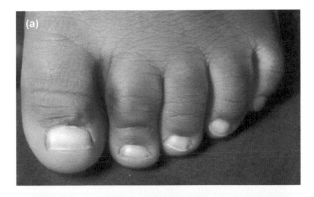

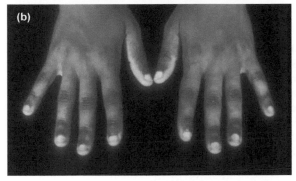

Figure 7.9a and b   Chilblains (perniosis), with reddish-purple lesions on the toes of a child, occurring several hours after exposure to the cold (7.9a). 7.9b shows chilblains on the hands of a woman of Afro-Caribbean origin. Chilblains may be painful or itchy and usually resolve in a few days.

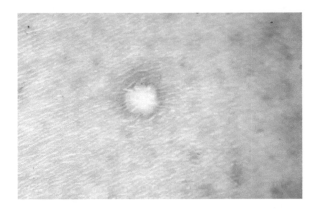

Figure 7.10   Malignant atrophic papulosis (Degos' disease), showing a small depressed porcelain white lesion with an elevated red border on the trunk. There may be many infarctive lesions on the skin with the subsequent development of similar lesions in the brain and gastrointestinal tract. Histology shows an atrophic epidermis, wedge-shaped infarct, and thrombosis of the vessels in the subcutaneous fat.

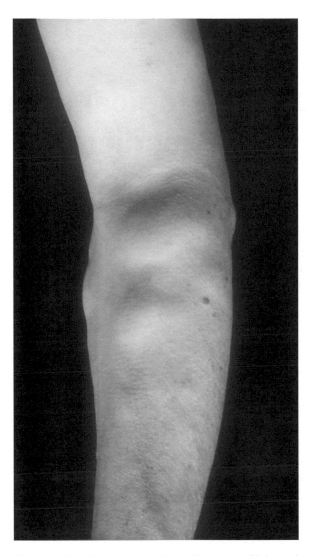

Figure 7.11   Lipomas may be solitary or multiple and are usually asymptomatic. 7.11 shows multiple lipomas on the arm in a patient in whom the soft lumps were symmetrical.

CHAPTER 8

Dermatological aspects of internal medicine

ACANTHOSIS NIGRICANS
AMYLOIDOSIS
Primary localized cutaneous amyloidosis
**Primary and myeloma-associated systemic
    amyloidosis**
AUTOIMMUNE AND CONNECTIVE TISSUE DISEASES
Lupus erythematosus
Dermatomyositis
Scleroderma

SARCOIDOSIS AND OTHER GRANULOMATOUS
DISORDERS
Sarcoidosis
Granuloma annulare
Necrobiosis lipoidica
MAST CELL DISORDERS
XANTHOMATOUS DISORDERS
OTHER METABOLIC OR NUTRITIONAL DISORDERS
Generalized pruritus

Some of the most interesting aspects of dermatology are seen when general internal medicine and dermatology overlap. Skin lesions may be part of a systemic disease, as occurs in sarcoidosis or systemic lupus erythematosus, or may be a manifestation of an underlying disease or process, as seen in acanthosis nigricans.

ACANTHOSIS NIGRICANS

Acanthosis nigricans, in which there is hyperpigmentation and hyperkeratosis of the flexures (e.g. a velvety appearance in the axillae), exists in two forms. In the absence of obesity, acanthosis nigricans may be an important clinical sign of an underlying adenocarcinoma, e.g. carcinoma of the stomach. The changes of acanthosis nigricans in younger obese patients, in which the nape of neck and antecubital fossae are often involved, are associated with insulin resistance (hyperinsulinaemia) and sometimes overt diabetes mellitus.

AMYLOIDOSIS

Amyloidosis occurs as primary localized cutaneous variants, including a papular form, lichen amyloidosus, and macular amyloid, and as systemic types of amyloidosis. Systemic amyloidosis includes those forms associated with plasma cell dyscrasia, either overt as in multiple myeloma, or undeclared as in 'primary' systemic amyloidosis, amyloidosis secondary to a number of chronic diseases, and some familial amyloidoses. Secondary amyloidosis occurs in chronic inflammatory diseases such as chronic infections, rheumatoid arthritis, and other forms of arthritis and connective tissue diseases.

Primary localized cutaneous amyloidosis

Several distinctive forms of primary localized cutaneous amyloidosis (PLCA) exist, and **lichen amyloidosus** and **macular amyloid** may coexist, suggesting a single pathological process. The papular form usually presents as an itchy eruption of discrete hyperkeratotic papules, scaly and often hyperpigmented, predominantly on the shins. In macular amyloisosis there are clusters of small pigmented macules, which may coalesce to produce macular hyperpigmented areas, sometimes with a 'rippled' pattern. There is also a nodular form of PLCA.

Primary and myeloma-associated systemic amyloidosis

Primary systemic amyloidosis often presents after the age of 60 years old with non-specific symptoms including fatigue, weight loss, shortness of breath, paraesthesiae, and hoarseness. Characteristic clinical features are carpal tunnel syndrome, macroglossia, signs of bleeding into the skin due to amyloid deposits in blood vessel walls, hepatomegaly, and oedema. Biopsy of the mucocutaneous lesions is often diagnostic using a Congo red stain or sometimes requiring electron microscopy. Periorbital purpura after proctoscopy and rectal biopsy as a diagnostic procedure ('post-proctoscopic palpebral purpura') is a memorable sign. An underlying plasma cell dyscrasia should be sought.

> **Therapeutic suggestions**
> Melphalan and oral corticosteroids

AUTOIMMUNE AND CONNECTIVE TISSUE DISEASES

The autoimmune diseases include **Addison's disease (adrenal insufficiency)** in which one sees melanin pigmentation of the buccal mucosa and skin, particularly the palmar creases. This may be associated with vitiligo (Chapter 10), alopecia areata (Chapter 3), and other autoimmune diseases, including pernicious anaemia and thyroiditis.

Immunological abnormalities have been demonstrated in the connective tissue diseases, which include various types of lupus erythematosus (LE), dermatomyositis, morphoea (localized and generalized), systemic sclerosis (systemic scleroderma), and graft-versus-host disease. Lupus erythematosus occurs as discoid LE, systemic LE, and subacute LE. Systemic sclerosis has been classified into diffuse cutaneous systemic sclerosis and limited cutaneous systemic sclerosis.

Lupus erythematosus

In **discoid LE**, erythematous atrophic plaques occur on sun-exposed areas, especially the face and scalp, where it may cause scarring alopecia. Discoid LE usually runs a chronic course and about 5–10% of cases progress to systemic LE. The diagnosis is confirmed by skin biopsy for histology and direct immunofluorescence (IMF) on lesional skin. The antinuclear antibody (ANA) may be positive in 20% of cases.

Involvement of the basal layer in LE often produces marked hyperpigmentation in black patients that may persist once the disease is inactive. Hyperpigmentation and hypopigmentation may occur together.

> **Therapeutic suggestions**
> Sunscreens
> Topical corticosteroids
> Antimalarials
>
> **Second-line treatment**
> Intralesional corticosteroids
> Oral retinoids

Systemic LE characteristically presents with an erythematous, macular 'butterfly' rash on the nose and cheeks. Other sun-exposed areas (e.g. the dorsa of the hands) may be affected and there is a female preponderance. Provoking factors include sunlight and drugs such as hydralazine, methyl dopa, isoniazid, and phenytoin. There may also be rheumatological, renal, cardiac, and haematopoietic symptoms and signs. Investigations should include skin biopsies for histology and/or direct IMF of lesional and non-lesional skin (the 'lupus band' test), an autoantibody screen, and assessment for systemic involvement. **Subacute LE** presents with lesions on sun-exposed areas, which are either annular in appearance, sometimes forming large polycyclic lesions, or comprise smaller papulosquamous lesions.

> **Therapeutic suggestions**
> Sunscreens
> Topical corticosteroids
> Antimalarials
>
> **Second-line treatment**
> Dapsone
> Thalidomide

Dermatomyositis

In dermatomyositis there is a reddish ('heliotrope') periocular rash usually accompanied by lesions on the dorsa of the hands and associated with proximal myopathy. A skin biopsy may reveal non-specific inflammatory changes. However, the plasma creatine kinase (CK) level is elevated. Electromyography (EMG) of affected muscles characteristically shows spontaneous fibrillation and polyphasic myopathic potentials. Muscle biopsy, if required, should be carried out on clinically abnormal muscle, on the opposite side, thus avoiding histological EMG changes. Magnetic resonance imaging (MRI) can detect areas of inflammatory myopathy.

Although the association between dermatomyositis and underlying malignancy has probably been overstated in the past, a limited search for the commoner forms of malignancy is advisable, particularly in the elderly.

> **Therapeutic suggestions**
> Oral corticosteroids
> Antimalarials
>
> **Second-line treatment**
> Oral immunosuppressive agents
> Intravenous immune globulin

Scleroderma

Sclerosis of the skin occurs in **morphoea**, which may be localized or rarely generalized, **diffuse cutaneous systemic sclerosis**, and **limited cutaneous systemic sclerosis**, previously known as CRST (CREST) syndrome. In morphoea, there may be localized sclerotic plaques accompanied by brown macular areas of skin (not necessarily atrophic), particularly on the trunk. The problem may be asymptomatic or accompanied by pruritus. Linear morphoea is well-known, particularly in children, and uncommonly sclerosis of the skin overlying limb joints may lead to developmental problems.

Morphoea and lichen sclerosus (lichen sclerosus et atrophicus, LSA) may coexist, LSA more commonly affecting the genital sites than the skin. In men the term balanitis xerotica obliterans (BXO) is sometimes used, but the disease is often not as severe as the name implies. The increased risk of neoplastic change in genital LSA is important to consider.

In diffuse cutaneous systemic sclerosis, there is loss of mobility of the skin and other organs due to fibrosis, leading to tight perioral skin with gastrointestinal and respiratory problems. The hand features of CREST syndrome (calcinosis, Raynaud's phenomenon, sclerodactyly, telangiectasia) and oesophageal dysfunction may occur in the limited cutaneous form or as part of diffuse cutaneous systemic sclerosis.

Therapeutic suggestions
Nifedipine
Intravenous prostaglandin E$_1$

Second-line treatment
Systemic methotrexate
Oral cyclophosphamide with corticosteroids

Investigation of autoantibodies in connective tissue diseases
Lupus erythematosus
ANA
Double-stranded DNA antibodies
Antibodies to ribonucleoprotein antigens
  Sm (Smith)
  U1 ribonucleoprotein (U1RNP)
  Ro (SSA) and La (SSB)
  Antiphospholipid antibodies*

Dermatomyositis
Antibodies to Jo-1

Scleroderma
Anticentromere antibodies

*Anticardiolipin and other antiphospholipid antibodies occur in 20% of SLE patients and are a feature of the **antiphospholipid syndrome**, including venous and arterial thromboses, strokes, migraine, and a history of recurrent spontaneous abortions. They should be measured in patients who present with livedo reticularis.

SARCOIDOSIS AND OTHER GRANULOMATOUS DISORDERS

The non-infectious granulomatous disorders include sarcoidosis, granuloma annulare, and necrobiosis lipoidica. Granulomatous diseases caused by bacterial infections (e.g. tuberculosis and leprosy) and fungal infections are discussed in Chapter 12.

Sarcoidosis

Skin lesions occur in about 30% of patients with systemic sarcoidosis, but cutaneous sarcoidosis can occur without systemic disease. Significant pulmonary disease may be asymptomatic and the extent of skin involvement does not correlate with the extent of systemic disease.

The specific skin lesions of sarcoidosis arise from a dense accumulation of epithelioid granulomas in the dermis or subcutis and can be of variable morphology. Erythema nodosum (Chapter 7) is a non-specific clinical feature of early or acute sarcoidosis without the characteristic sarcoidal granulomas. Nodular sarcoid lesions are often annular and reddish-brown or violaceous in colour. There may be multiple papules and larger plaques, particularly on the nose, a site at which the skin changes are frequently perniotic in appearance (lupus pernio). Skin lesions can affect pre-existing scars (the Koebner or isomorphic phenomenon), sometimes referred to as scar sarcoidosis. A rare but characteristic telangiectatic form of sarcoidosis, angiolupoid sarcoid, affects women, almost always on the sides of the nasal bridge, on the adjacent cheek, or below the eyebrows. Sometimes the nodular lesions are solely subcutaneous, and erythrodermic and lichenoid sarcoidosis are unusual morphological forms.

Sarcoidosis is more common in black skin and in African-Americans typical lesions include annular lesions on the nose, hypopigmented macules and papules, keloid-like lesions, ulcerative, verrucous, and large nodular forms. Erythema nodosum is uncommon in black skin. In white skin the colour of the lesions ranges from yellowish to the livid violaceous colour which is most marked in lupus pernio. The epidermis is rarely affected and scarring is unusual except in the papular and annular forms.

Sarcoid-like reactions in a scar should be distinguished from a foreign body reaction. A granulomatous sarcoidal reaction to any pigment of a tattoo may occur, either alone or accompanied by other signs of sarcoidosis.

Investigation of sarcoidosis*

Skin biopsy

Chest X-ray

Angiotensin-converting enzyme (ACE)

Blood calcium level

ECG

ESR or viscosity

Full blood count (anaemia, leukopenia)

Gammaglobulins (increased in 50%)

Pulmonary function tests

Computed tomography of the chest

Hand X-rays

*The most specific investigation was the Kveim test, in which sarcoidal tissue from the spleen of an affected individual was injected intradermally to produce an epithelioid cell granulomatous reaction. A positive response was the development of a reddish papule at 2–3 weeks. Excision at 6 weeks showed the confirmatory histology. However, this test is no longer used because of the infective risk of injecting human tissue.

Therapeutic suggestions

Topical corticosteroids

Intralesional corticosteroids

Oral corticosteroids

Antimalarials

Second-line treatment

Methotrexate

Minocyline

Doxycycline

Oral isotretinoin

Granuloma annulare

Granuloma annulare (GA) is a reaction pattern in the skin with a well-established morphology and natural history. **Localized GA** is the commonest form and presents as reddish collections of papules which form annular lesions, with palpable edges, often over the knuckles and on the elbows. Other areas of the skin may be involved and a diffuse or generalized pattern occurs uncommonly. In **generalized GA**, there are numerous skin-coloured or erythematous slightly palpable coalescing papules, arranged symmetrically on the trunk and limbs. Annular lesions may be violaceous in colour and itching is often a feature of the generalized form. **Perforating** (referring to extrusion of material through the epidermis) and **subcutaneous GA** are uncommon patterns, the latter sometimes being difficult to distinguish from rheumatoid nodules.

It is reasonable to exclude diabetes mellitus in patients with GA but this probably occurs in only about 5% cases of localized GA, rising to up to 20% in the generalized form. The distinction from necrobiosis lipoidica, more strongly associated with diabetes mellitus, is usually made histologically but GA and necrobiosis lipoidica can occur in the same patient. The sporadic occurrence of GA and its tendency to remit spontaneously makes it difficult to assess the efficacy of treatment and in many cases no treatment is needed.

Therapeutic suggestions

Topical corticosteroids

Cryotherapy

Second-line treatment

Intralesional corticosteroids

PUVA

Necrobiosis lipoidica

Necrobiosis lipoidica occurs as reddish-yellow shiny plaques on the shins, with atrophy and telangiectasia, but early lesions are less obvious. Lesions may ulcerate and a chronic course is usual. In most cases, lesions are bilateral, and they are similar in appearance whether occurring in diabetic or non-diabetic patients.

The association of diabetes mellitus in up to 60% patients who have necrobiosis lipoidica was probably overestimated in previous studies of tertiary referral populations. Necrobiosis lipoidica may precede the development of diabetes in about one in 10 individuals. It can occur at any age, but usually develops in young adults and in early middle age. Only about 0.3% patients with diabetes mellitus will have necrobiosis lipoidica.

Therapeutic suggestions
Topical corticosteroids with polythene occlusion
Intralesional corticosteroids

Second-line treatment
Nicotinamide
Clofazimine

MAST CELL DISORDERS

The mastocytoses can involve the skin in a number of ways. **Urticaria pigmentosa** is a generalized form of cutaneous mastocytosis which may be macular, papular, or telangiectatic (**telangiectasia macularis eruptiva perstans**). Occasionally mast cell infiltration produces a diffuse yellow thickening of the skin. Single or multiple **mastocytomas** occur quite commonly in childhood mast cell disease but are unusual in adults.

Systemic mastocytosis, with involvement of the skeleton and gastrointestinal tract, may or may not be symptomatic, and the development of anaemia on an annual full blood count warrants further investigation. Mast cell leukaemia (malignant mastocytosis) is rare.

Therapeutic suggestions
Antihistamines

Second-line treatment
PUVA
UVA1 phototherapy
Topical corticosteroids with polythene occlusion
Interferon-alpha

XANTHOMATOUS DISORDERS

Xanthomatous lesions are usually associated with abnormal lipid metabolism and sometimes with specific types of hyperlipoproteinaemia. There are various types of xanthoma, including **eruptive xanthomas**, **tuberous xanthomas**, **tendon xanthomas**, and **plane xanthomas**. **Xanthelasmas** are flat yellowish lesions on the eyelids. In addition there are some rare forms of xanthomatous diseases such as **necrobiotic xanthogranuloma**, which is associated with systemic lesions and a monoclonal gammopathy.

OTHER METABOLIC OR NUTRITIONAL DISORDERS

Cutaneous manifestations of systemic diseases may also reflect nutritional status (e.g. scurvy), predominantly affect the dermis or vasculature (Chapters 6 and 7), or may be referred to as disorders of altered reactivity (Chapter 9).

Generalized pruritus

Itching without any obvious primary skin disease may be a presenting feature of an underlying systemic disorder. A full blood count may reveal polycythaemia vera, an important cause of itching after exposure to water (aquagenic pruritus). Iron deficiency, even in the absence of anaemia, can cause generalized pruritus. One should therefore check the serum ferritin and preferably iron-binding capacity, even if the haemoglobin is normal.

Liver biochemistry may demonstrate cholestasis, for example, due to mechanical obstruction of bile flow. It is worth checking an autoimmune profile, particularly in middle-aged women, considering primary biliary cirrhosis. Pruritus due to uraemia is usually associated with other features of renal failure. Serum urea and electrolytes and creatinine are simple screening tests and there may be secondary hyperparathyroidism.

Both hyper- and hypothyroidism may underlie generalized pruritus. Diabetes mellitus is associated with an increased incidence of genital itching only. Occasionally generalized pruritus will be the presenting symptom of a lymphoma, sometimes detectable on chest X-ray. In postmenopausal pruritus, typically associated with hot flushes, plasma follicle-stimulating hormone (FSH) and luteinizing hormone (LH) may be elevated.

FURTHER READING

Bolognia JL, Jorrizzo JL, Rapini RP, et al (eds). Dermatology. Philadelphia: Mosby, 2003.

Burns T, Breathnach S, Cox N, Griffiths C (eds). Rook's Textbook of Dermatology, 7th edn. Oxford: Blackwell Science, 2004.

Lovell CR. General laboratory investigations. In: Cerio R, Archer CB (eds). Clinical Investigation of Skin Disorders. London: Chapman and Hall Medical, 1998.

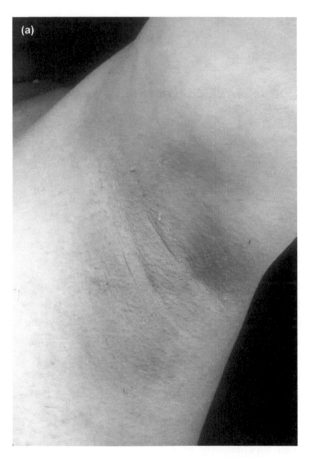
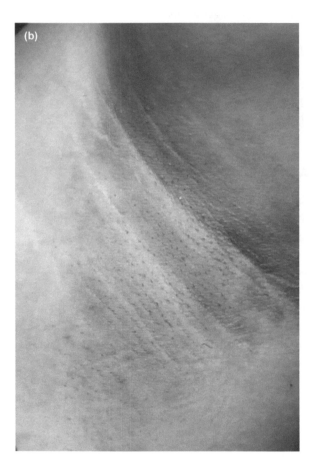

Figure 8.1a and b   Acanthosis nigricans, showing hyperpigmentation and hyperkeratosis of the axillary skin. Although this clinical appearance can herald the occurrence of an underlying adenocarcinoma, it is a relatively common sign of hyperinsulinaemia and sometimes frank diabetes mellitus in obese patients (8.1b).

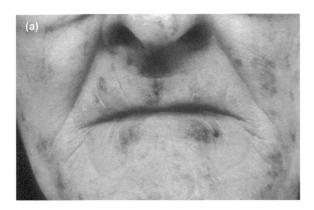

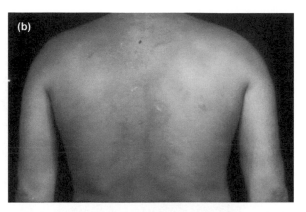

Figure 8.2a and b   Amyloidosis, with haemorrhagic perioral lesions in an elderly man with primary systemic amyloidosis (8.2a). Primary localized cutaneous variants include the papular form, lichen amyloidosus (8.2b), and macular amyloid, more common in Asians, which may be rather subtle and misdiagnosed as post-inflammatory hyperpigmentation.

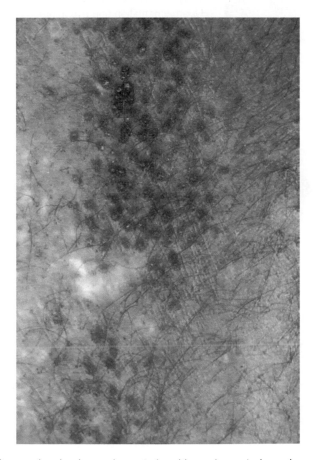

Figure 8.3   Lichen amyloidosus, showing hyperpigmented and hypopigmented papules on the shin of a black man.

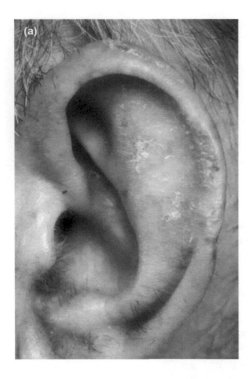

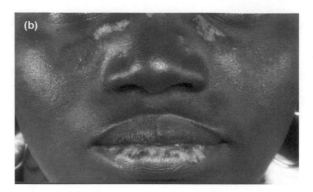

Figure 8.4a and b   Discoid lupus erythematosus. The ears are commonly involved in discoid lupus erythematosus (8.4a), a disorder exacerbated by sun exposure. (8.4b) Hyperpigmentation and hypopigmentation on the cheeks in a young woman of Afro-Caribbean origin, in whom the lower lip is also affected.

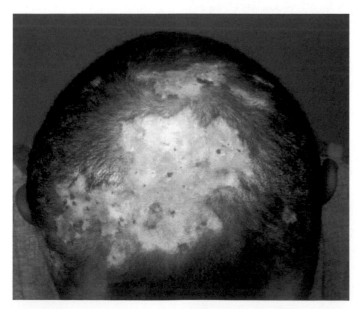

Figure 8.5   Discoid lupus erythematosus, a cause of scarring alopecia. The erythematous inflammatory component is readily seen, and the diagnosis confirmed by biopsy of an active area with direct immunofluorescence of lesional skin.

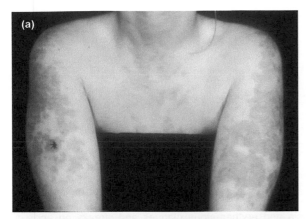

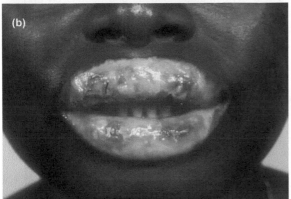

Figure 8.6a and b Systemic lupus erythematosus, showing macular erythematous lesions on sun-exposed sites (8.6a). 8.6b shows an inflammatory cheilitis in a young black child with systemic lupus erythematosus.

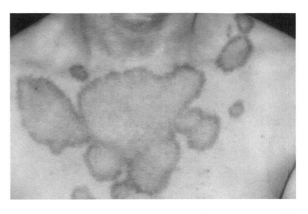

Figure 8.7 Subacute lupus erythematosus, with characteristic polycyclic annular lesions on the upper chest. The lesions are macular here but are sometimes papulosquamous, usually occurring on sun-exposed sites.

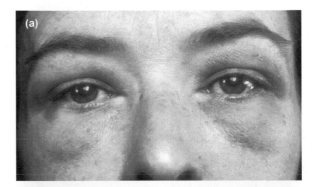

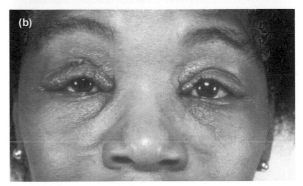

Figure 8.8a and b Dermatomyositis, showing periocular oedematous heliotrope lesions in a woman with proximal muscle weakness (8.8a). In black skin (8.8b) the oedematous nature of the lesions is a more useful clinical sign than their colour.

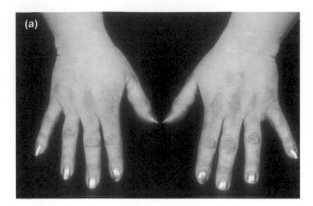

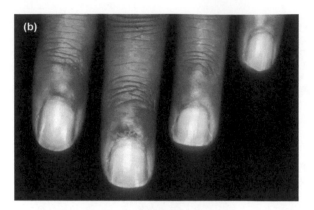

Figure 8.9a and b   Dermatomyositis, with nail-fold telangiectasia and erythematous plaques and streaks on and between the knuckles (8.9a). 8.9b shows hyperpigmentation at the site of the nail-fold changes in a black patient. The skin changes on the hands in dermatomyositis can sometimes be difficult to distinguish from those in lupus erythematosus.

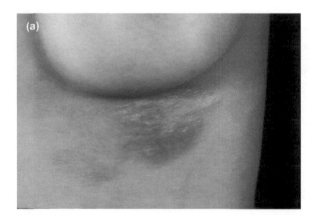

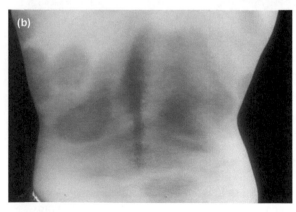

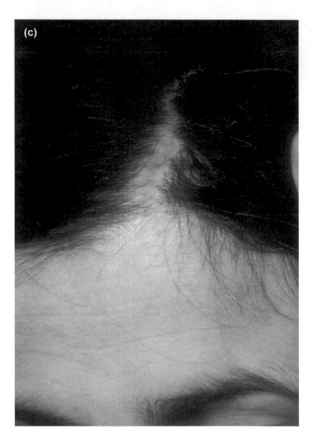

Figure 8.10a, b, and c   Localized morphoea, showing sclerosis of the skin with brown discoloration beneath the breast (8.10a) and light brown annular lesions on the back (8.10b). These brown patches are sometimes atrophic. (8.10c) A linear sclerotic lesion on the scalp ('en coup de sabre'). Morphoea can also be generalized but confined to the skin or part of a systemic process (diffuse cutaneous systemic sclerosis).

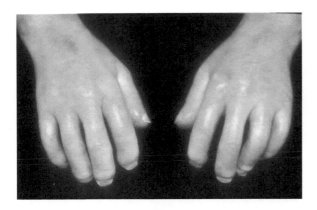

Figure 8.11 Primary cutaneous systemic sclerosis, showing diffuse shiny tight skin on the hands. Other areas of the skin were affected in this patient. Collagen accumulation and fibrosis leads to loss of mobility of the skin and other organs, including the gastrointestinal and respiratory tracts, although this is not always progressive.

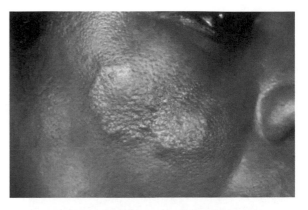

Figure 8.12 Sarcoidosis, with an annular plaque on the cheek of an Afro-Caribbean woman. Cutaneous sarcoidosis is more common in black skin.

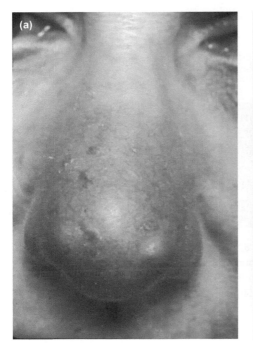

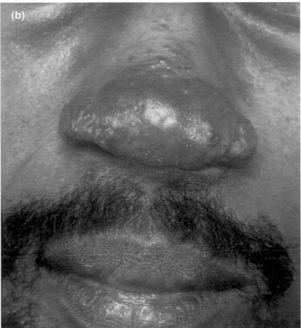

Figure 8.13a and b Sarcoidosis, showing violaceous lesions on the nose in a white man (8.13a) and in a man of Afro-Caribbean origin (8.13b). The term lupus pernio is often used for lesions on the nose.

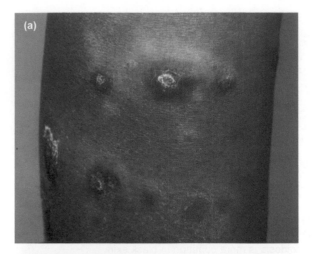

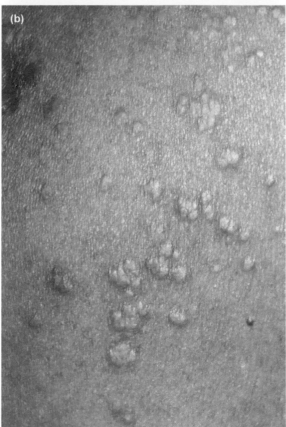

Figure 8.14a and b   Sarcoidosis, with nodular lesions on the arm in a patient with black skin (8.14a). 8.14b shows the unusual clinical pattern of lichenoid sarcoidosis on the lower back of a West Indian woman.

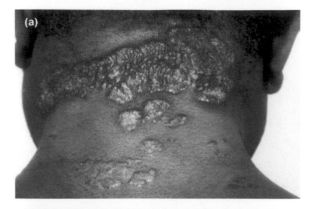

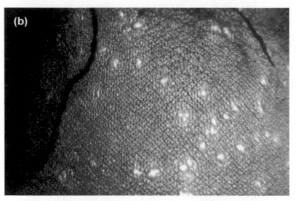

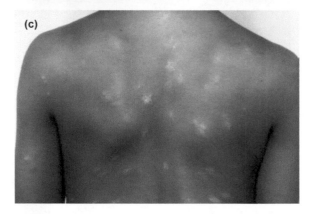

Figure 8.15a, b, and c   Sarcoidosis. Other variants of cutaneous sarcoidosis include hypertrophic sarcoidosis, seen on the nape of the neck (8.15a), papular sarcoidosis (8.15b), and hypopigmented forms, as shown in 8.15b and c.

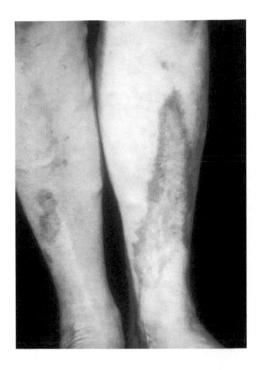

Figure 8.16 Necrobiosis lipoidica, showing reddish-yellow atrophic plaques on the shins. The dermal blood vessels become clearly visible and plaques may ulcerate. Many cases are associated with diabetes mellitus at the time of presentation and necrobiosis lipoidica can precede the development of diabetes mellitus.

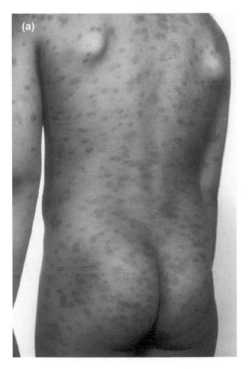

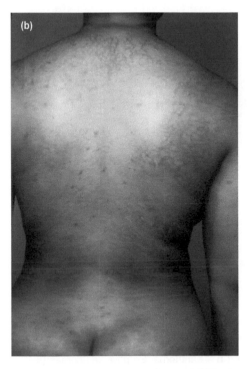

Figure 8.17a and b Urticaria pigmentosa. In black skin the distribution of the lesions of urticaria pigmentosa is characteristic. Individual lesions are hyperpigmented (8.17a) and close inspection of the skin may reveal telangiectatic lesions (8.17b).

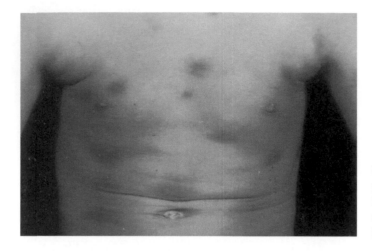

Figure 8.18 Mastocytoma. Although urticaria pigmentosa occurs in children, it is more common to see solitary or multiple mastocytomas, as shown in a child of Asian origin, in whom these benign tumours are hyperpigmented.

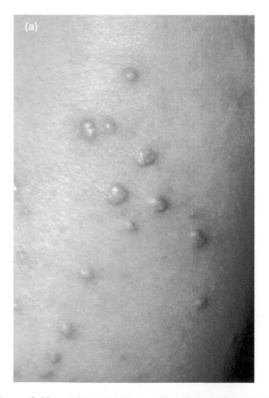

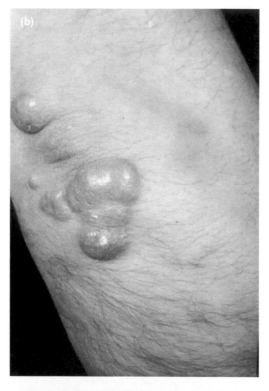

Figure 8.19a and b   Xanthoma. Eruptive xanthomas (8.19a) are usually multiple reddish-yellow lesions on the buttocks, arms, and legs. In white people the yellow colour can be better appreciated if the skin is stretched. Tuberous (tendon) xanthomas are nodular lesions, commonly occurring on the elbows (8.19b). The possibility of hyperlipoproteinaemia should be investigated. Associated systemic diseases include diabetes mellitus, hypothyroidism, pancreatitis, and nephrotic syndrome.

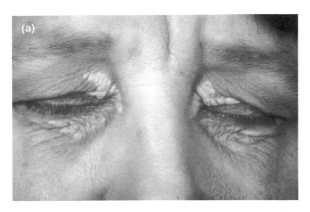

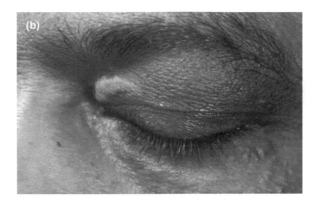

Figure 8.20a and b Xanthelasma, showing flat yellowish lesions on the eyelids (8.20a). The yellow colour is less obvious in deeply pigmented skin (8.20b).

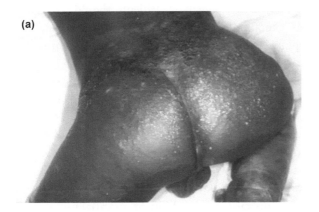

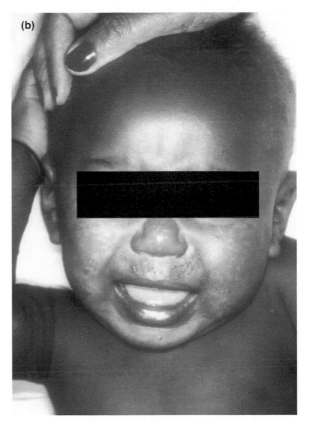

Figure 8.21a and b Acrodermatitis enteropathica, showing perianal (8.21a) and extensive perioral erosive lesions (8.21b) in a malnourished, zinc-deficient African child.

CHAPTER 9

Disorders of altered reactivity

URICARIA AND ANGIOEDEMA
Investigation of urticaria and angioedema
POLYMORPHIC ERUPTION OF PREGNANCY
DRUG REACTIONS

PHOTOSENSITIVE DISEASES
OTHER DISORDERS OF ALTERED REACTIVITY
Behçet's disease

Many dermatological diseases may be considered to be disorders of altered reactivity, in which the skin responds abnormally to a variety of stimuli, involving either immune or non-immune mechanisms. For example, altered immunological mechanisms are involved in the pathogenesis of allergic contact dermatitis, atopic dermatitis (Chapter 2), and vasculitis (Chapter 7), whereas dermographism is an example of an altered response to a physical stimulus.

Included in this section are the urticarias, drug reactions, the photodermatoses, **graft-versus-host disease**, and less well-defined disorders such as **annular erythema, Sweet's syndrome, eosinophilic cellulitis** (Wells' syndrome), and Behçet's disease. The overlap of these disorders with internal medicine is readily apparent.

URTICARIA AND ANGIOEDEMA

There is usually a typical history of recurrent itchy erythematous swellings (papules and wheals) due to leakage of the interstitial fluid from the blood vessels into the skin. **Chronic urticaria** by definition lasts for longer than 6 weeks, and in many cases no trigger is detected (**chronic idiopathic urticaria**). Urticaria can be mediated by a type I immunological reaction, as seen when a patient is **allergic** to a particular food or drug. Commonly reported ingestants include shellfish, strawberries, nuts, food additives, and

drugs, especially penicillin. Patients should avoid drugs containing aspirin, codeine, ibuprofen, and morphine, which can exacerbate urticaria by mast cell degranulation.

Stimuli which can induce the **physical urticarias** include **pressure** (**dermographism** or **delayed pressure urticaria**), **heat, cold**, and rarely **sunlight. Heat urticaria** may be localized or associated with **cholinergic urticaria**, which can be induced by exercise. **Contact urticaria** results from direct contact of the stimulus with the skin. Urticarial lesions persisting for 24 hours raise the possibility of urticarial vasculitis, which is sometimes associated with systemic lupus erythematosus.

Therapeutic suggestions
Non- or low-sedating antihistamine
Addition of sedative antihistamine
Addition of intermittent oral corticosteroids

Second-line treatment
Ciclosporin
Azathioprine

Patients may present with urticaria and deeper subcutaneous oedema (angioedema) in which breathing may be threatened due to swelling of the throat and tongue. Angioedema is often idiopathic, and **idiopathic angioedema** may sometimes be familial. Other forms include drug-induced angioedema and, uncommonly, hereditary angioedema (HAE) in its various forms.

Angiotensin-converting enzyme (ACE) inhibitors are often overlooked as a cause of angioedema but are currently responsible for most cases of acute angioedema seen in Emergency Departments. **ACE inhibitor-induced angioedema** is not associated with urticaria and continued administration of the drugs tends to lead to more severe attacks. The incidence of ACE inhibitor-induced angioedema is more common in African-Americans than in white patients.

The differential diagnosis includes **HAE** in its various forms, in which C1 esterase inhibitor deficiency causes an overproduction of bradykinin rather than ACE inhibitor-induced decreased degradation. HAE may be accompanied by a transient red rash but is not associated with urticaria.

Investigation of urticaria and angioedema

No routine blood tests are necessary in most patients with chronic urticaria. A full blood count to look for eosinophilia as a sign of a parasitic infection may be useful in patients returning from abroad. A plasma viscosity and erythrocyte sedimentation rate (ESR) may be elevated. A RAST may occasionally confirm a clinical suspicion of a specific allergic trigger. When angioedema and urticaria occur together, the cause of the angioedema is usually not HAE, but when there is a positive family history, one should check the serum complement C4 is used as a screening test. It is recommended that the C1 esterase inhibitor levels be measured only when the C4 is decreased, since falsely low levels of C1 esterase inhibitor have been recorded when blood samples are not assayed promptly.

Hyperthyroidism may present as symptomatic dermographism. In patients with unexplained urticaria, an oral challenge test battery may reveal unexpected triggers, such as salicylates and benzoates, but these investigations are no longer routinely performed because of low positive yields.

POLYMORPHIC ERUPTION OF PREGNANCY

Cutaneous eruptions seen during pregnancy are often urticarial in nature. Polymorphic eruption of pregnancy (pruritic urticarial papules and plaques of pregnancy, PUPP) is common, presenting with itching and the development of reddish urticarial papules and plaques, usually during the third trimester. The lesions often begin on the abdomen and later involve the thighs, buttocks, and arms.

Polymorphic eruption of pregnancy, unlike pemphigoid gestationis (herpes gestationis) (Chapter 5), does not show subepidermal bullae histologically and direct immunofluorescence (IMF) is negative. Pruritus is a common symptom in pregnancy and is sometimes associated with cholestasis.

> **Therapeutic suggestions**
> Topical corticosteroids
> Oral antihistamines
>
> **Second-line treatment**
> Oral corticosteroids

DRUG REACTIONS

Drug reactions may occur as a result of non-immunological mechanisms (e.g. overdose, side effects, drug interactions) or, less commonly, because of an immunological, allergic response to the drug itself, a metabolite of the drug, or to a contaminant of the drug. Autoimmune reactions may also occur.

Recognized patterns of drug rashes include exanthematic (maculopapular) reactions, purpura, annular erythema, exfoliative dermatitis, anaphylaxis and anaphylactoid reactions, urticaria, erythema multiforme, Stevens–Johnson syndrome and toxic epidermal necrolysis, fixed drug eruptions, lichenoid drug eruptions, photosensitivity, pigmentation reactions, vasculitis, lupus erythematosus-like syndrome, dermatomyositis reactions, scleroderma-like reactions, and erythema nodosum.

The clinical features of toxic erythema (reactive erythema) may be seen in the absence of a drug, and the causative agent is usually presumed to be viral.

Common causative agents include penicillins, sulphonamides, and non-steroidal anti-inflammatory drugs. In the absence of reliable objective tests for drug allergies, the diagnosis is usually made following a careful history. Oral challenge with the suspected drug is often considered to be unwise in case of a serious systemic reaction.

PHOTOSENSITIVE DISEASES

Photosensitivity is relatively common. Some of the idiopathic photodermatoses are considered likely to be allergic in origin, ultraviolet (UV) radiation inducing a delayed hypersensitivity reaction. The photodermatoses include polymorphic light eruption, juvenile spring eruption, actinic prurigo, chronic actinic dermatitis (a form of chronic photosensitive eczema), **hydroa vacciniforme**, actinic reticuloid, and **solar urticaria.**

Polymorphic (polymorphous) light eruption (PLE) affects 10–15% of the population and is more common in women. **Juvenile spring eruption**, affecting the ears of children (usually boys), is thought to be a mild transient form of PLE.

Actinic prurigo is an itchy photosensitivity disorder in children, occasionally persisting or beginning in adult life. Excoriated lesions affect sun-exposed sites, sparing covered areas, but may occur on the lower back and buttocks.

Chronic actinic dermatitis (CAD) is an uncommon severe photosensitive eczema which predominantly affects elderly men. Patients may not notice that sun exposure exacerbates the rash. Severe lichenified eczema affects the face, the nape of the neck, V of the chest, and backs of hands. A sharp cut-off is seen at the collar line and cuffs (Chapter 2).

Light-protected areas under the chin and behind the ears are spared. If the patient becomes erythrodermic, these signs may be obscured. CAD should be included in the differential diagnosis of erythroderma and air-borne contact dermatitis.

Actinic reticuloid is a form of cutaneous lymphoma that represents the most severe end of the photosensitive eczema/chronic actinic dermatitis disease spectrum.

Drug-induced photosensitive rashes can be phototoxic or photoallergic, and may be induced by topical or systemic agents. Phototoxic reactions depend on a direct interaction of UV radiation or visible light with the drug or chemical in the skin, without an allergic reaction. Examples include psoralens, used therapeutically for PUVA therapy and contained in some plants, which may produce a phytophotodermatitis. Drug-induced photoallergy is much less common and difficult to prove. Chlorpromazine, sulphonamides, and possibly thiazides may lead to both phototoxic and photoallergic reactions.

Investigation of photosensitive rashes
PLE
Skin biopsy (routine histology, direct IMF)
Autoantibodies, including ANA, Ro/SSA, La/SSB
Photoprovocation tests

Photosensitive eczema
Patch and photopatch tests

CAD
Monochromator tests

Photosensitivity may reflect underlying metabolic, genetic, or nutritional diseases such as certain types of porphyria, **xeroderma pigmentosum**, and **pellagra.**

The main **cutaneous porphyrias** are porphyria cutanea tarda (PCT), erythropoietic protoporphyria, and variegate porphyria. Patients develop sun-induced skin fragility, with blistering on the dorsa of the hands and other light-exposed areas, milia formation, and hypertrichosis, commonly on the forehead. The diagnosis is confirmed by measuring appropriate porphyrins in the blood, urine and/or faeces.

In PCT, alcohol-induced liver damage occurs to a variable extent, and management measures include minimization of sun exposure, reduced alcohol intake, antimalarial therapy, and venesection.

In addition, some diseases may be exacerbated by sun exposure. These include lupus erythematosus, rosacea, Darier's disease, Grover's disease, herpes simplex, and occasionally psoriasis following sunburn (the isomorphic or Koebner phenomenon).

Therapeutic suggestions
PLE
Sun-avoidance measures
Sunscreens

Second-line treatment
Oral corticosteroids
PUVA
Narrow-band UVB
UVB

CAD
Photoprotection
Emollients
Topical corticosteroids

Second-line treatment
Azathioprine

OTHER DISORDERS OF ALTERED REACTIVITY

Graft-versus-host-disease (GVHD) occurs when lymphoid cells from an immunocompetent donor are introduced into a histoincompatible recipient incapable of rejecting them. Moderate to severe acute GVHD affects up to 35%, and the incidence of chronic GVHD, appearing after 3 months, is up to 50%.

In acute GVHD a generalized erythematous morbilliform rash is accompanied by fever, a malar flush, and redness of the palms. In chronic GVHD the initial eruption is usually lichenoid. Hyper- or hypopigmentation are often prominent features and the process can be generalized or localized.

Erythema annulare centrifugum (EAC) is a characteristic annular erythema in which a small pink infiltrated papule slowly enlarges to form a ring, as the central area flattens and fades. Lesions are often up to 8 cm diameter, either with a smooth surface or with slight scaling behind the advancing edge. In black skin the erythema is not apparent and one sees annular areas of hyperpigmentation with slight scaling.

Sweet's syndrome is characterized by fever, peripheral blood leukocytosis (neutrophilia), acute onset of painful erythematous papules, plaques or nodules, and histological findings of dense neutrophilic infiltrate, in the absence of primary vasculitis. Sweet's syndrome is often idiopathic but it may be drug-induced, and it is important to consider the possibility of an underlying malignancy, which may or may not be haematological (e.g. there may be a leukaemia or paraproteinaemia).

Therapeutic suggestions
Oral corticosteroids
Topical corticosteroids

Second-line treatment
Indometacin
Colchicine

Eosinophilic cellulitis (Wells' syndrome) is rare and presents with single or multiple itchy erythematous plaques with features resembling urticaria and cellulitis. The diagnosis is confirmed by the histological finding of 'flame figures'.

Aphthous ulcers, usually occurring on the lip, tongue, or buccal mucosa, are common in healthy individuals but the prevalence is reported to be increased in celiac disease. Apthous ulceration can also be a cause of great discomfort in patients with Behçet's syndrome.

> **Therapeutic suggestions**
> Topical corticosteroids
> Oral tetracycline
> Antimicrobial mouth rinses

Behçet's disease

Behçet's disease is a multisytem disease that is defined by the presence of oral aphthosis with at least two of the following: genital aphthae, synovitis, posterior uveitis, cutaneous pustular vasculitis, or meningoencephalitis, in the absence of inflammatory bowel disease or autoimmune diseases. It typically affects young adults and is uncommon in northern Europe and the USA, but common in Middle Eastern and Japanese populations.

The diagnosis of Behçet's disease should be suspected in any patient with recurrent and extensive oral aphthosis. Other causes of aphthosis such as inflammatory bowel disease, as well as lesions that mimic aphthae such as herpes simplex virus infection, must be excluded. The diagnosis should also be considered in young patients with deep vein thrombosis, particularly in the absence of other risk factors or thrombophilia. A positive pathergy provocation test, read at 24–48 hours, may further support the diagnosis.

> **Therapeutic suggestions**
> Topical corticosteroids
> Intralesional corticosteroids
>
> **Second-line treatment**
> Colchicine
> Dapsone
> Thalidomide

FURTHER READING

Bolognia JL, Jorrizzo JL, Rapini RP, et al (eds). Dermatology. Philadelphia: Mosby, 2003.

Burns T, Breathnach S, Cox N, Griffiths C (eds). Rook's Textbook of Dermatology, 7th edn. Oxford: Blackwell Science, 2004.

Murphy GM. Investigation of allergic skin disorders and the photodermatoses. In: Cerio R, Archer CB (eds). Clinical Investigation of Skin Disorders. London: Chapman and Hall Medical, 1998.

(a)
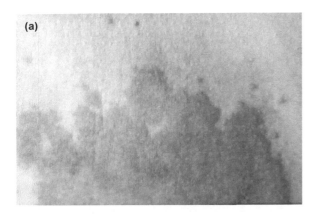

(b)
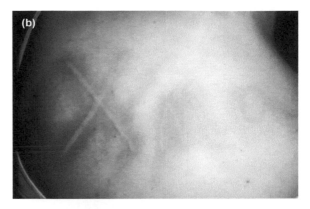

Figure 9.1a and b Urticaria, showing red raised itchy transient wheals (9.1a). No obvious trigger factor is found in about 50% of cases. The timing of the urticarial reaction may point to an allergy to foods, e.g. shellfish, strawberries, nuts, or food additives. Dermographism may be part of other forms of urticaria or may occur alone as symptomatic dermographism (factitious urticaria). (9.1b) Prominent wheal and flare responses to a dermographometer in a young woman who presented to a December clinic.

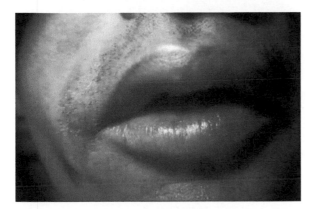

Figure 9.2 Angioedema (angioneurotic oedema), showing prominent swelling of the lips. Subcutaneous swelling usually affects the face, tongue, and larynx and, in severe cases, laryngeal oedema can lead to respiratory obstruction.

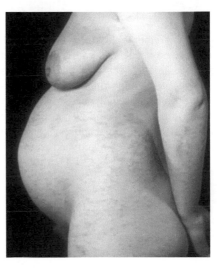

Figure 9.3 Polymorphic eruption of pregnancy (pruritic urticarial papules and plaques of pregnancy, PUPP), showing itchy red urticated lesions on the abdomen, buttocks, thighs, and arms.

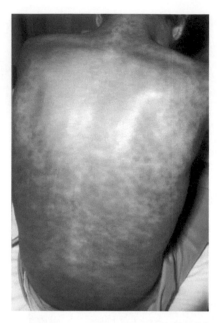

Figure 9.4 Toxic erythema (reactive erythema). This clinical picture may be associated with a viral or bacterial illness or uncommonly with malignancy. The term 'reactive erythema' is perhaps preferable to 'toxic erythema' since the eruption is not necessarily due to a toxin. 9.4 shows a dusky red ampicillin eruption, commonly seen in patients with infectious mononucleosis, and not necessarily implying an allergy to penicillin.

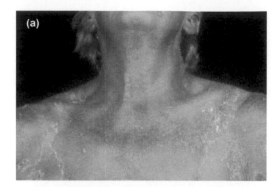

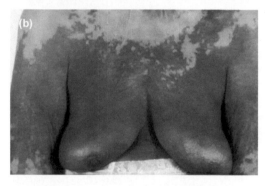

Figure 9.5a and b Exfoliative dermatitis, showing erythroderma and desquamation (9.5a), and prominent desquamation and hypopigmentation in a black woman (9.5b). This clinical picture is seen in drug reactions, atopic dermatitis, allergic contact dermatitis, psoriasis, and lymphoma.

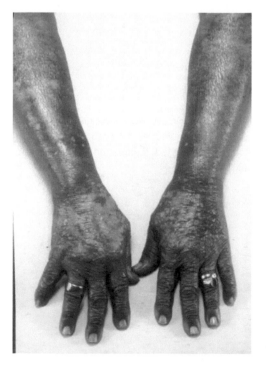

Figure 9.6 Lichenoid drug eruption, occurring on the forearms and dorsa of the hands in a patient with black skin.

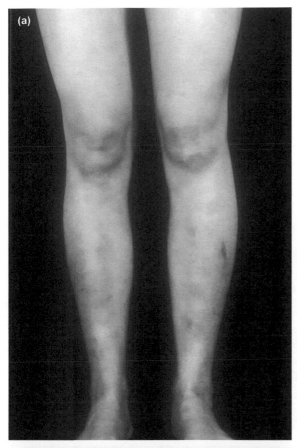

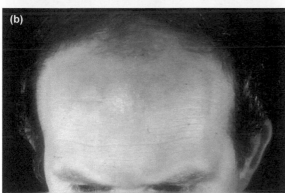

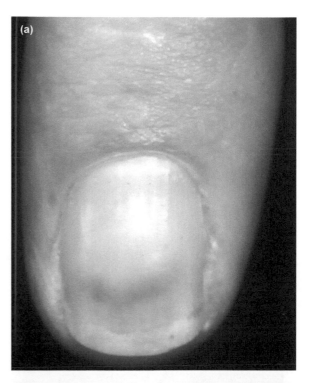

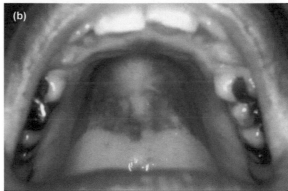

Figure 9.8a and b   Antimalarial pigmentation, showing prominent dusky blue pigmentation of the subungual region (9.8a) and palate (9.8b).

Figure 9.7a and b   Drug-induced pigmentation. (9.7a) Prominent bruise-like bluish pigmentation on the shins caused by minocycline, a response more common in the elderly, probably related to increased blood vessel fragility, since marked minocycline-induced pigmentation has been seen in a concurrent user of potent topical corticosteroids (CB Archer, personal observation). (9.7b) The slate-blue pigmentation caused by amiodarone, in which the pigment lipofuscin is deposited in the dermis of light-exposed areas.

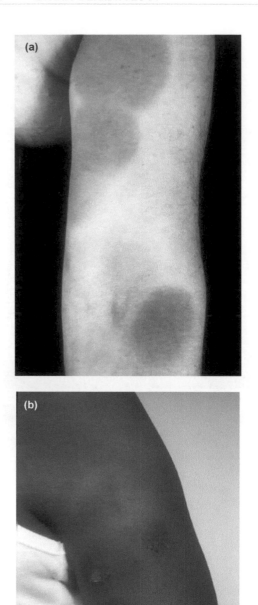

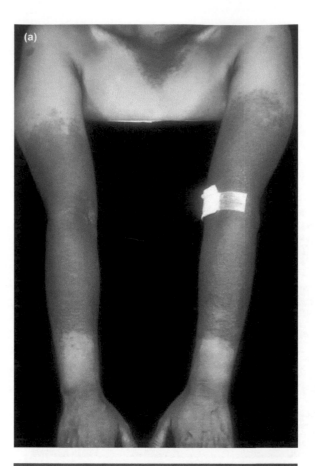

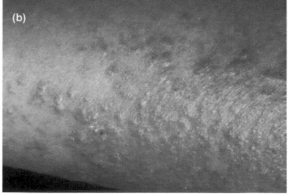

Figure 9.9a and b   Fixed drug eruption. 9.9a shows prominent hyperpigmentation, which is also seen on the upper arm of a patient with black skin (9.9b).

Figure 9.10a and b   Polymorphic (polymorphous) light eruption (PLE), showing a marked confluent erythematous rash on the arms and V of the neck in a young woman (9.10a). 9.10b shows the polymorphic nature of the eruption, with itchy papules and plaques on the sun-exposed surface of the arm. The face is often spared.

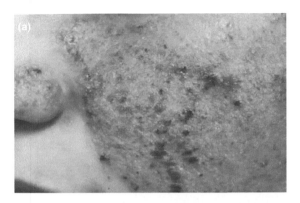

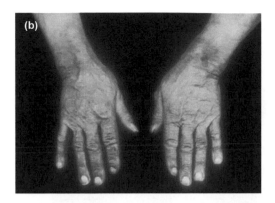

Figure 9.11a and b   Chronic actinic dermatitis (photosensitive eczema) is more frequently seen in men, the eczematous eruption involving the face (9.11a), nape of the neck, and dorsa of the hands (9.11b). There is a spectrum of disease severity, with lymphoma at one end of the spectrum (actinic reticuloid).

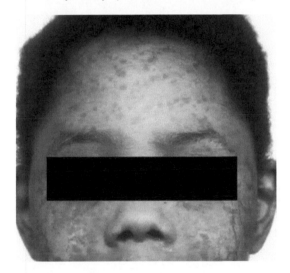

Figure 9.12   Hydroa vacciniforme, a rare disorder of childhood, resulting in depressed scarring of the face and, in this child, post-inflammatory hyperpigmentation. Some lesions are arranged in a linear pattern as a result of scratching.

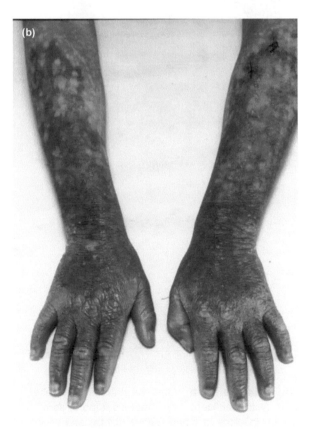

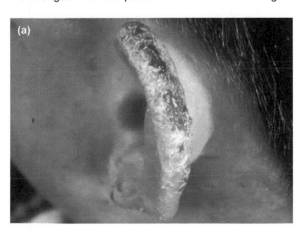

Figure 9.13 a and b   Rothmund–Thomson syndrome is arare genetic disease in which the skin is photosensitive. 9.13ashows marked ulceration of the outer helix of the ear and 9.13bshows hyperpigmentation and hypopigmentation on the handsand forearms in a person with deeply pigmented skin.

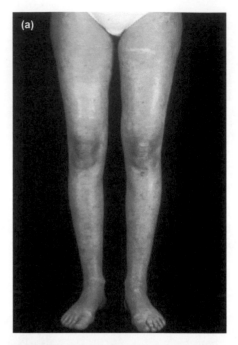

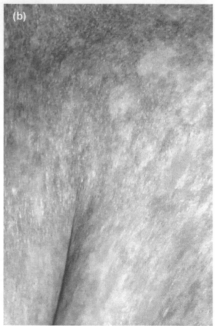

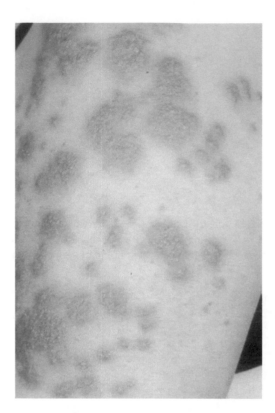

Figure 9.15 Sweet's syndrome (acute febrile neutrophilic dermatosis), showing reddish raised infiltrated lesions on the upper arm. Sweet's syndrome is usually accompanied by fever and an elevated peripheral blood neutrophil count, but these features can be more transient than the skin lesions and may therefore be missed.

Figure 9.14a and b Graft-versus-host disease (GVHD), with confluent erythematous ('morbilliform') lesions on the legs in acute GVHD (9.14a) and widespread hyperpigmented lesions on the shoulder region in chronic GVHD (9.14b). GVHD occurs after transplant operations when immunologically competent donor lymphocytes react with the skin. Lichenoid lesions are often seen in the chronic form of the disease.

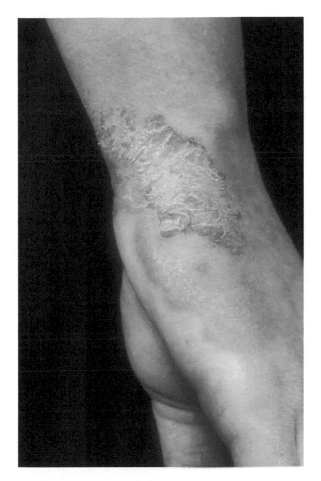

Figure 9.16 Eosinophilic cellulitis (Wells' syndrome), showing an erythematous plaque on the wrist and hand. The clinical presentation is variable and the diagnosis is confirmed by the histological finding of 'flame figures'.

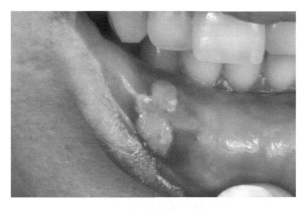

Figure 9.17 Aphthous ulceration, showing two painful ulcers on the mucosal surface of the lower lip. Other sites include the tongue and buccal mucosa. Aphthous ulcers are common in healthy individuals but the incidence is increased in coeliac disease.

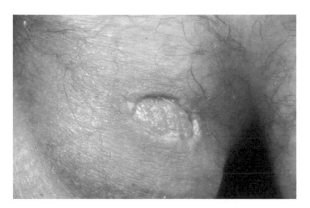

Figure 9.18 Behçet's disease, showing a prominent punched-out ulcer on the scrotum. The diagnosis of Behçet's syndrome should be suspected in any patient with recurrent and extensive oral aphthosis.

CHAPTER 10

Disorders of melanocytes

DISORDERS OF PIGMENTATION
Decreased or absent pigmentation
Increased pigmentation

BENIGN MELANOCYTIC NAEVI
ATYPICAL NAEVI
MALIGNANT MELANOMA

Disorders of skin pigmentation may be due to primary abnormalities of melanocyte structure and function, as in vitiligo, or may reflect secondary changes associated with other skin diseases, as one sees in post-inflammatory hyperpigmentation and post-inflammatory hypopigmentation in, for example, psoriasis and atopic dermatitis (Chapter 1). The mechanism of decreased pigmentation is different in pityriasis versicolor (Chapter 12). In addition, collections of naevus cells occur in benign melanocytic naevi and in the various types of malignant melanoma.

DISORDERS OF PIGMENTATION

Decreased or absent pigmentation

Vitiligo affects about 1% of the population, is more common in females than in males, occurs at any age (peak incidence 20–35 years old), and is commonly familial. Macular areas of depigmentation, sometimes with preceding hypopigmentation, tend to be symmetrical and are susceptible to sunburn, due to an absence of melanocytes. Vitiligo can be socially and psychologically devastating in patients with deeply pigmented skin and is a significant problem in white skin, especially in the summer months when the vitiliginous skin may become sunburnt and the vitiligo more noticeable as the surrounding skin becomes suntanned.

Vitiligo may be associated with alopecia areata, pernicious anaemia, thyroiditis, and Addison's disease

(adrenal insufficiency), consistent with an autoimmune pathogenesis.

> **Therapeutic suggestions**
> Topical corticosteroids
> Topical tacrolimus
> Cosmetic camouflage
>
> **Second-line treatment**
> Narrow-band UVB
> PUVA

Albinism is a rare group of congenital disorders in which melanin synthesis is decreased or absent, leading to changes in the skin, eyes, and hair. The number of melanocytes is normal but melanogenesis is impaired or absent due to defective tyrosinase activity. Patients are at an increased risk of developing skin cancers related to excessive solar damage.

The term **poliosis** refers to localized depigmentation of hair. It may affect the scalp hair, eyelashes, eyebrows, or body hair and may be associated with vitiligo, alopecia areata, tuberous sclerosis, and the congenital abnormality **piebaldism**.

Idiopathic guttate hypomelanosis, characterized by groups of small hypopigmented and depigmented macules, is common, particularly on sun-exposed surfaces. My preferred term for the type associated with chronic sun exposure in white skin is 'actinic guttate hypomelanosis' (personal view, CB Archer, 2007). This seems different from that occasionally seen in young people with deeply pigmented skin. The distinction of idiopathic guttate hypomelanosis from vitiligo is sometimes difficult clinically but the number of melanocytes is often normal (as opposed to being absent in vitiligo), there being an impairment of keratinocyte melanization.

Hypomelanosis of Ito (incontinentia pigmenti achromians) is a rare disease in which linear whorled or streaked hypopigmented macules are seen, usually in early childhood.

Chemical leukoderma, initially an industrial problem, can be utilized therapeutically. The monobenzyl ether of hydroquinone induces irreversible depigmentation in patients with extensive vitiligo, and hydroquinone reversibly damages melanocytes, being routinely used in skin 'lightening' creams and lotions.

Post-inflammatory hypopigmentation is common in suntanned white patients and may be seen in black patients with the inflammatory skin diseases of psoriasis and atopic dermatitis. However, in black patients post-inflammatory hyperpigmentation is more common (Chapter 1).

Increased pigmentation

Melasma (chloasma) is more common in women, particularly but not exclusively affecting those who are pregnant or taking a combined (oestrogen-containing) oral contraceptive. Brown pigmentation occurs on the face, especially the cheeks, forehead, and the upper lip region, but covered sites can also be affected. Melasma may resolve or persist after delivery of the baby or discontinuation of the oral contaceptive.

Therapeutic suggestions
Tretinoin/hydroquinone/corticosteroid
   combination
Tretinoin
Adapalene

Second-line treatment
Azelaic acid
Kojic acid

Becker's naevus is an acquired, large, light or dark brown, usually hair-bearing, lesion, occurring on the shoulder or chest region of young men. It is generally unilateral and histologically there is thickening of the epidermis with an increased number of melanocytes and basal cell layer hyperpigmentation.

Café au lait macules are light or dark brown macules, usually a few centimetres in diameter, occurring on the trunk and sometimes other areas of the body. Isolated lesions occur in about 10% of the population but multiple café au lait spots should raise the suspicion of an underlying systemic disorder, such as generalized neurofibromatosis (Chapter 6) or **Albright's syndrome**; the latter comprises polyostotic fibrous dysplasia, café au lait macules, precocious puberty in females, and endocrine abnormalities.

Melanin deposition is also seen on mucosal surfaces such as the lips, glans penis, and vulva, when the term mucosal **melanosis** is used. Penile melanosis refers to lesions without lentiginous hyperplasia, and is different from post-inflammatory hyperpigmentation as occurs in lichen planus or lichen sclerosus et atrophicus (LSA).

Incontinentia pigmenti is an X-linked genetic disease, presenting with blisters in a whorle-like pattern and later results in whorled hyperpigmentation. Other forms of hyperpigmentation include **erythema dyschromicum perstans** (ashy dermatosis), **reticulate pigmentary anomaly of the flexures**, **ochronosis** (Chapter 1), and hyperpigmentation induced by the topical or systemic administration of metals (**argyria**, silver; **chrysiasis**, gold). As discussed in Chapter 4, ashy dermatosis may be a variant of lichen planus pigmentosus.

Post-inflammatory hyperpigmentation particularly occurs in diseases which affect the basal layer of the epidermis, such as lichen planus and lupus erythematosus, when melanin spills over into the upper dermis to be engulfed by macrophages (pigmentary incontinence). The common inflammatory dermatoses psoriasis and atopic dermatitis account for many cases of post-inflammatory hyperpigmentation in black skin. As discussed in Chapter 1, the hyperpigmentation in deeply pigmented patients can persist well after the active disease process has subsided and sometimes indefinitely.

BENIGN MELANOCYTIC NAEVI

Benign melanocytic naevi arise from epidermal melanocytes, usually in childhood, and are subdivided into **junctional, compound** (with epidermal and dermal components), and **intradermal** types. It is thought that as a junctional naevus matures, melanocytes pass into the dermis forming a compound naevus, resulting, after a number of years, in an entirely intradermal naevus.

A **halo naevus**, usually occurring on the trunk of children or young adults with a surrounding area of depigmentation, is often a sign of impending resolution of the naevus. Halo naevi are often multiple and can occur independently of vitiligo, the depigmentation resulting from immunologically mediated melanocytic damage.

In children, the histology of benign melanocytic naevi can resemble malignant melanoma, particularly in a **Spitz naevus (juvenile melanoma)**. This reddish-brown lesion often occurs on the face or limbs. **Naevus spilus** is a benign melanocytic naevus with a speckled clinical appearance, sometimes referred to as a speckled naevus.

A large **congenital giant hairy pigmented naevus** has both an epidermal and dermal component and is associated with a low risk of malignant change, usually being excised therefore during puberty. There are a number of other types of congenital naevi. Linear **epidermal naevi** are common. **Sebaceous naevi**, usually seen on the scalp, have a low potential for the development of associated basal cell carcinomas and are probably best excised at some stage, usually in early adulthood.

Localized increased numbers of dermal melanocytes occur in blue naevi, including Mongolian spots, common blue naevi, and in naevus of Ota and naevus of Ito. The colour of a blue naevus is due to the appearance of the deep dermal melanin when viewed through overlying structures such as blood vessels. **Mongolian spots** are common congenital lesions, almost a normal finding in black or Asian babies, typically occurring as diffuse blue-grey macules on the lower back or buttocks. There is a presumed incomplete migration of melanocytes from the neural crest to the epidermis in foetal life. Regression by the teenage years is usual but some blue naevi persist indefinitely.

Common blue naevi are usually raised dome-shaped blue lesions, particularly occurring on the limbs, and often presenting to the dermatologist in early adulthood.

The **naevus of Ota** affects the cheek (in the distribution of the trigeminal nerve), is usually present at birth and unilateral, particularly occurring in black patients and those of Japanese origin. A similar dermal process is seen in the **naevus of Ito**, which affects the skin on the upper trunk.

Other benign pigmented lesions include lentigos (lentigines) and seborrhoeic keratoses (Chapter 11).

Benign lentigos are usually light brown in colour and may be congenital or acquired. Solar lentigos (a preferred term to senile lentigos) occur after prolonged sun exposure on the hands, face, and upper back. Histological studies have shown that on the face, solar lentigos may gradually evolve into seborrhoeic keratoses, and the clinical distinction between the two can be difficult.

ATYPICAL NAEVI

Atypical naevi are usually defined as being at least 5 mm in diameter, with an irregular shape and irregular colour. They may be solitary naevi (in up to 16% of the normal population) or, less commonly, may occur as part of the **atypical naevus syndrome** phenotype, a more worrying situation, in terms of the increased risk of developing malignant melanoma, when there is a positive family history of malignant melanoma.

The specificity of clinicopathological findings in atypical naevi is controversial and the term 'dysplastic' used here may be misleading and not the same as when used to describe a progression towards neoplasia, as one sees in cervical dysplasia or in the skin with the actinic keratosis – intraepidermal carcinoma – squamous carcinoma spectrum. The melanocytes exhibit cytological atypia, accompanied by the architectural features of melanocytic hyperplasia, often continuous along the junctional zone and sometimes producing bridging between rete pegs. There is often a stromal reaction with increased vascularity, stromal condensation, and a lymphohistiocytic response. However, some of these features have been seen in banal melanocytic naevi.

MALIGNANT MELANOMA

There was a steady increase in the incidence of malignant melanoma of the skin from 1950 to the mid-1990s. Since 1995 there has been a stabilization of the annual incidence in women of all ages. However, the incidence continues to increase in men, particularly older men. Superficial spreading and nodular melanomas tend to occur in the 20–60-year-old age group, whilst lentigo maligna melanoma mostly affects those over the age of 60 years old.

Factors associated with increased risk for an individual include the total number of benign melanocytic naevi (>100 naevi), a skin type that easily sunburns, and excessive sun exposure, particularly repeated episodes of sunburn (although this is debatable). The atypical or dysplastic naevus syndrome is accepted as a risk factor, but in the absence of a family history of malignant melanoma, the increased risk from the presence of sporadic atypical naevi in the presence of multiple banal melanocytic naevi is considered to be only a little greater than for multiple benign melanocytic naevi per se.

Four main variants of malignant melanoma are seen:

- superficial spreading melanoma
- nodular melanoma
- lentigo maligna melanoma
- acral lentiginous melanoma.

Superficial spreading malignant melanoma accounts for about 50% of melanomas in the UK,

and is more common in women, particularly on the lower leg. Nodular melanoma in seen in about 25% of melanomas in the UK, and is more common in men, especially on the trunk. **Lentigo maligna** (Hutchinson's melonotic freckle) occurs as a macular variably pigmented intraepidermal process on the face of elderly white patients. After many years, a lentigo maligna may develop palpable and deeper components, when it is referred to as a lentigo maligna melanoma, i.e. a nodular melanoma arising in a lentigo maligna. Acral lentiginous melanoma particularly affects the palms, soles, and nail beds, and may be diagnosed relatively late. It accounts for about 10% of all melanomas in white patients but over 50% of melanomas in darker-skinned races. Occasionally a melanoma may be non-pigmented or amelanotic, and the distinction from a squamous carcinoma or pyogenic granuloma is important.

Malignant melanomas often arise on normal-appearing skin but in around 30% there is histological evidence of a benign melanocytic naevus. As discussed in Chapter 1, a history of changes in a long-standing naevus may be an important sign of development of a malignant melanoma. In considering superficial spreading melanoma, one may use the ABCD mnemonic, in which A = asymmetry, B = irregular border, C = irregular colour, and D = diameter >1 cm. There is also a seven-point checklist devised from research based in Glasgow, in which there are three major and four minor features:

Major features:
1. Change in size
2. Change in shape
3. Change in colour

Minor features:
1. Diameter >5 mm
2. Inflammation
3. Oozing or bleeding
4. Mild itch or altered sensation

The presence of one major feature in an adult would probably lead to excision of the pigmented lesion, and the presence of additional minor features should increase clinical suspicion.

Prognosis largely depends on the depth of the tumour, so that early recognition is important. The **Breslow thickness** (in millimetres) is measured from the granular layer of the epidermis to the deepest tumour cells. Histopathological reports of malignant melanoma also refer to the **Clark's level**, reflecting horizontal or vertical growth phases.

A Breslow thickness of ≤1 mm is associated with a 5-year survival rate of greater than 95%, whereas a tumour thickness of 3–3.5 mm is associated with a 5-year survival rate of around 50%. For this reason, there has been great emphasis on early recognition of new or changing pigmented lesions in public information programmes. An in-situ superficial spreading melanoma may be excised with a 2–5 mm margin.

Ulceration is an additional and independent poor prognostic sign, and a high mitotic count and presence of tumour cells in vessels are poor prognostic signs.

Therapeutic suggestions
Wide excision
Selective lymph node excision

Second-line treatment
Immunotherapy
Isolated limb perfusion
Chemotherapy

FURTHER READING

Bolognia JL, Jorrizzo JL, Rapini RP, et al (eds). Dermatology. Philadelphia: Mosby, 2003.

Burns T, Breathnach S, Cox N, Griffiths C (eds). Rook's Textbook of Dermatology, 7th edn. Oxford: Blackwell Science, 2004.

Gawkrodger DJ. Dermatology: An Illustrated Colour Text, 3rd edn. Edinburgh: Churchill Livingstone, 2002.

Harper J, Oranje A, Prose N (eds). Textbook of Paediatric Dermatology, 2nd edn. Oxford: Blackwell Science, 2006.

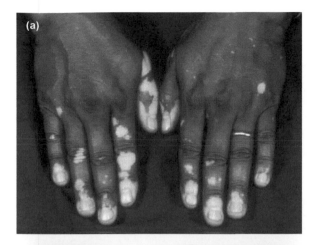

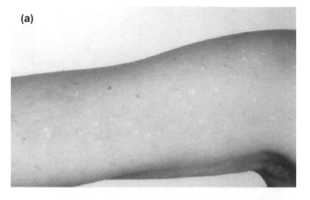

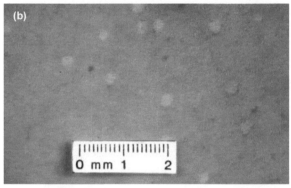

Figure 10.2a and b Idiopathic guttate hypomelanosis on the upper arm of a white patient (10.2a) and on the trunk in deeply pigmented skin (10.2b). Vitiligo sometimes presents with guttate lesions in which hypopigmentation precedes depigmentation.

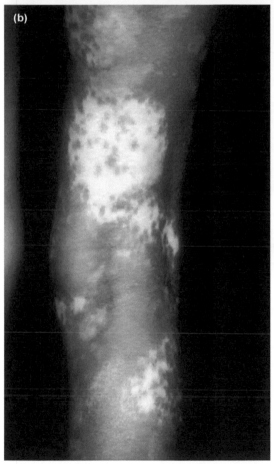

Figure 10.1a and b Vitiligo, with symmetrical areas of depigmentation on the hands (10.1a) and very noticeable depigmentation on the posterior aspect of the leg in a black man (10.1b). Islands of normal pigment can be seen within the depigmented areas.

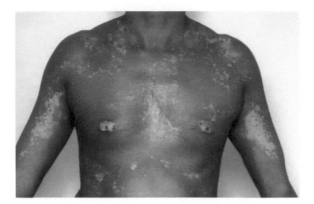

Figure 10.3 Vitiligo, after treatment with PUVA in a man with deeply pigmented skin, showing areas of repigmentation within the erythematous areas of vitiligo. The depigmented skin of vitiligo is susceptible to sunburn and use of sunscreens can prevent this and further tanning of the surrounding normal skin.

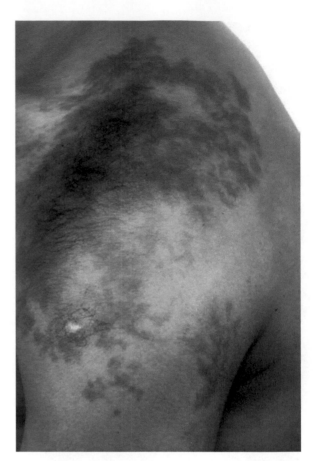

Figure 10.5 Becker's naevus, showing a dark brown lesion on the shoulder of a young man with deeply pigmented skin. Usually no treatment is required apart from reassurance.

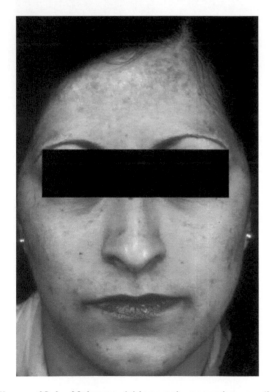

Figure 10.4 Melasma (chloasma), occurring on the face, particularly the forehead, in a woman of Indian origin. The hyperpigmentation may also affect non-sun-exposed sites and may be persistent. If associated with pregnancy or an oestrogen-containing oral contraceptive, the pigmentation often resolves once the source of oestrogen has been removed.

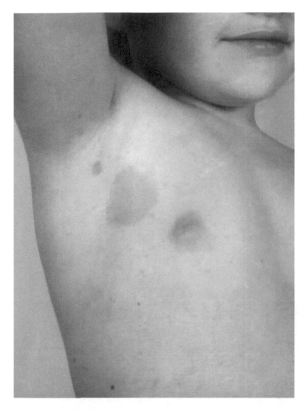

Figure 10.6 Café au lait macules may occur as a normal variant or as part of a systemic disorder such as neurofibromatosis, as seen on the trunk of a young girl. The presence of axillary freckling may help to confirm a diagnosis of type 1 neurofibromatosis.

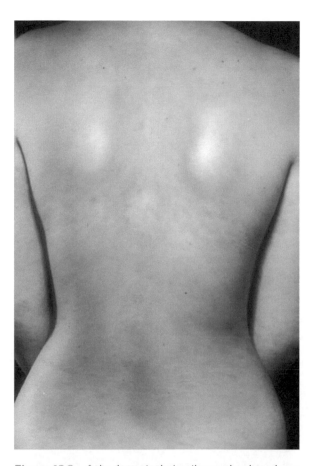

Figure 10.8 Ashy dermatosis (erythema dyschromicum perstans), showing slate-grey macules on the lower back of a patient with deeply pigmented skin. This clinical entity is well recognized in South America, being of uncertain aetiology. In other parts of the world it is regarded as a macular variant of lichen planus pigmentosus (Chapters 1 and 4).

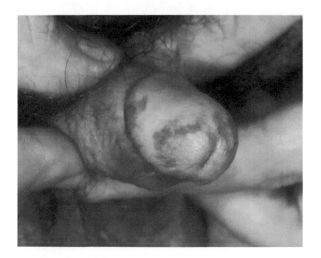

Figure 10.7 Melanosis, affecting the glans penis. Other mucosal sites include the lips and vulva.

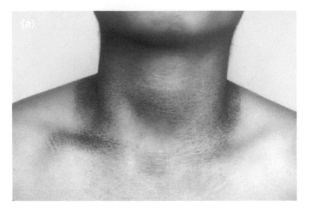

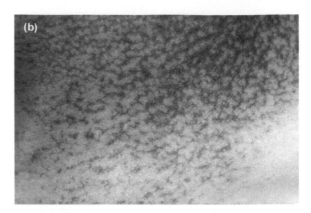

Figure 10.9a and b   Reticulate pigmented anomaly of the flexures (Dowling–Degos disease), showing characteristic pigmentation on the neck and upper chest (10.9a). 10.9b is a close-up view of the reticulate pattern of pigmentation. Common sites include the flexures, inner thighs, neck, scrotum, face, and scalp. Histology shows epidermal budding in a filiform pattern.

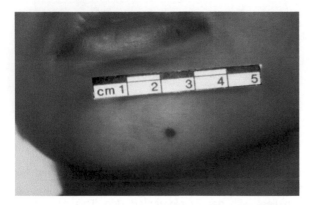

Figure 10.10   Benign melanocytic naevus on the chin of a child with deeply pigmented skin.

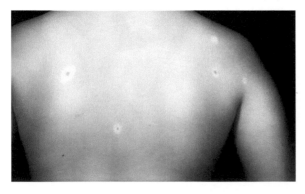

Figure 10.11   Halo naevi on the back, showing zones of depigmentation surrounding benign melanocytic naevi. The naevus on the right shoulder has undergone spontaneous resolution. The patient did not have vitiligo elsewhere.

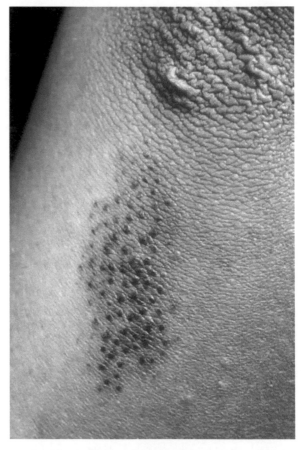

Figure 10.12   Naevus spilus, showing a collection of dark brown lesions forming a large speckled naevus near the elbow in a person with deeply pigmented skin.

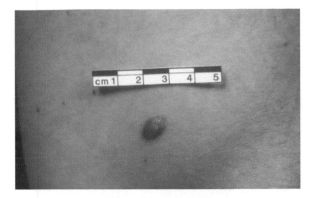

Figure 10.13   Spitz naevus (juvenile melanoma), showing a reddish-brown regular-shaped lesion on the upper arm of a child. The face and trunk are also common sites for this benign lesion which gradually turns brown. A Spitzoid malignant melanoma is rare.

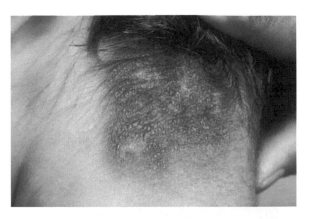

Figure 10.15   Epidermal naevus, showing a deeply pigmented lesion in the occipital region. The surface change reflecting the epidermal nature of the lesion can be seen.

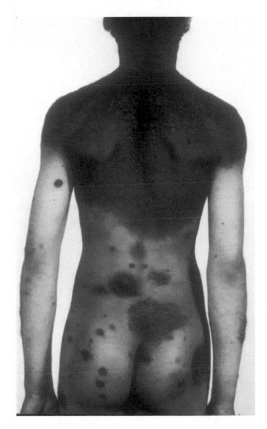

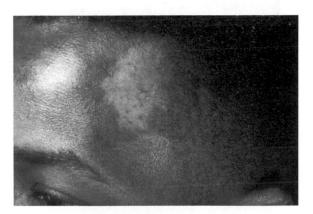

Figure 10.16   Congenital naevus, showing a hypopigmented naevus near the left temple in a young man of Afro-Caribbean origin.

Figure 10.14   Congenital giant hairy pigmented naevus. This extensive naevus affects the scalp, upper back, the trunk, and buttocks of a boy with deeply pigmented skin. Large congenital pigmented naevi are considered to be at risk of subsequent development of malignant melanoma, and are best excised if feasible.

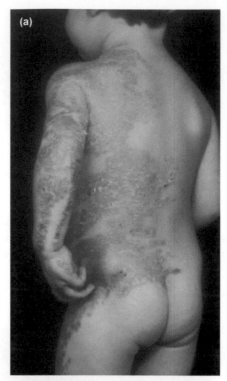

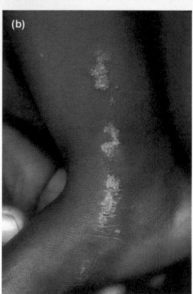

Figure 10.17a and b   Inflammatory linear verrucous epidermal naevus (ILVEN). 10.17a shows an extensive inflammatory naevus on the left side of the body and in 10.17b the linear nature is readily apparent, although in deeply pigmented skin, the inflammatory component is not seen. Extensive epidermal naevi may be part of the epidermal naevus syndrome, also comprising various skeletal, neurological, and ocular abnormalities.

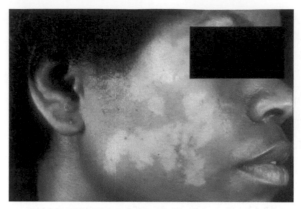

Figure 10.18   Hypopigmented naevus. In deeply pigmented people, congenital naevi are frequently hypopigmented or depigmented (achromic), as seen on the cheek of this Afro-Caribbean woman.

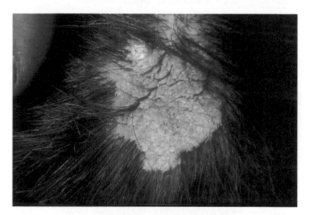

Figure 10.19   Sebaceous naevus, showing a warty lesion on a child's scalp. Occasionally a basal carcinoma will develop during puberty and sebaceous naevi are therefore usually excised in the teenage years.

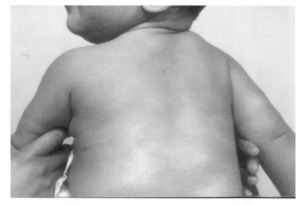

Figure 10.20   Blue naevus (Mongolian spot), due to deep dermal melanin pigmentation in a child of Afro-Caribbean origin. These lesions are common in black skin.

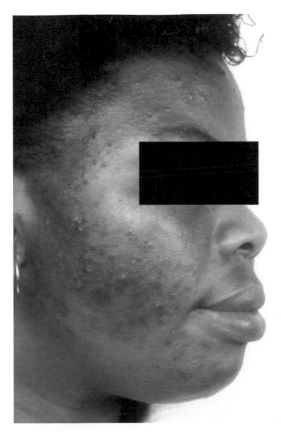

Figure 10.21   Naevus of Ota, showing unilateral diffuse bluish/dark brown lesions on the cheek. The naevus of Ota is more commonly seen in black patients or those of Japanese origin.

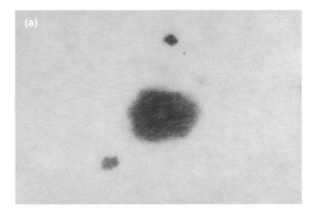

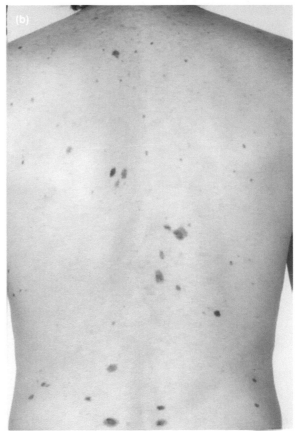

Figure 10.22a and b   Atypical naevus (dysplastic naevus), showing a brown naevus on the trunk, greater than 5 mm in diameter and with irregular pigmentation and shape (10.22a). These are sometimes multiple (10.22b) and require particular attention if there is a family history of malignant melanoma. The original clinicopathological definition of dysplastic naevus is frequently less rigidly applied and the term 'atypical naevus syndrome' is preferred to 'dysplastic naevus syndrome'.

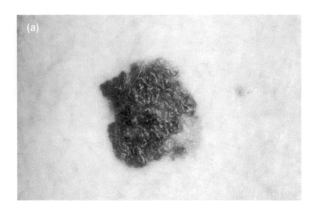

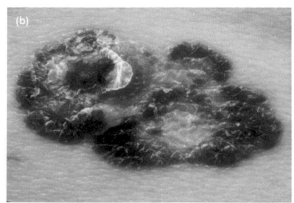

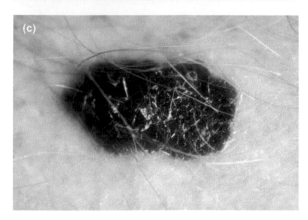

Figure 10.23a, b, and c   Superficial spreading malignant melanoma. (10.23a) A long-standing naevus on the trunk in which the light brown pigmentation rapidly became blackened. The edge of the lesion is irregular. (10.23b) A larger superficial spreading malignant melanoma on the back with irregular pigmentation and a pink raised component. (10.23c) A black superficial spreading malignant melanoma.

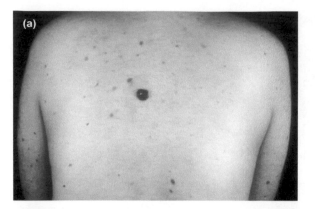

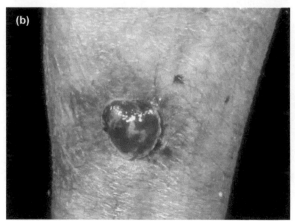

Figure 10.24a and b   Nodular malignant melanoma, showing a large pigmented lesion on the back of a white man with numerous other benign melanocytic naevi (10.24a). 10.24b shows a fleshy nodular melanoma on the lower leg of a white woman.

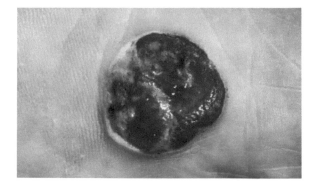

Figure 10.25   Nodular malignant melanoma, showing an amelanotic tumour on the palm of the hand. Amelanotic malignant melanoma is important to distinguish from a rapidly developing pyogenic granuloma (Chapter 6), emphasizing the need for histological confirmation.

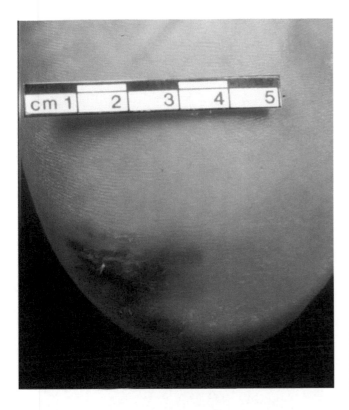

Figure 10.26   Acral lentiginous melanoma, showing a diffuse pigmented lesion on the heel of the foot. Such lesions may have been present for some time before the patient seeks medical advice.

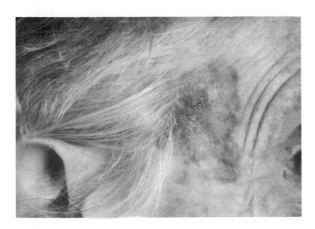

Figure 10.27   Lentigo maligna (Hutchinson's freckle) affecting the right temple region of an elderly woman. The area of darker pigmentation raises the suspicion that this lesion is not merely a benign solar lentigo. The natural history of lentigo maligna is variable and the lesion may remain unchanged for many years, but in all but the very elderly, excision is advisable.

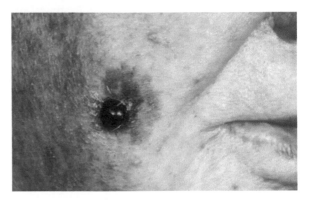

Figure 10.28   Lentigo maligna melanoma, showing a black nodular melanoma developing in a long-standing lentigo maligna (Hutchinson's freckle) on the right cheek. Once the nodular component has developed, the prognosis is similar to that of a nodular malignant melanoma of the same depth (Breslow thickness) on histology.

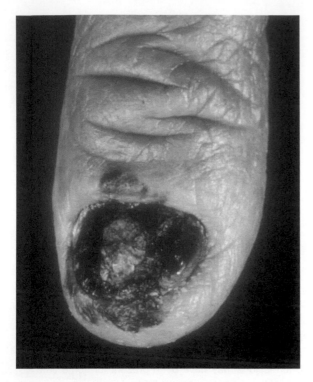

Figure 10.29 Subungual malignant melanoma. These tumours develop from the nail-fold region (Hutchinson's sign) and may be amelanotic. Late presentation is associated with a poor prognosis.

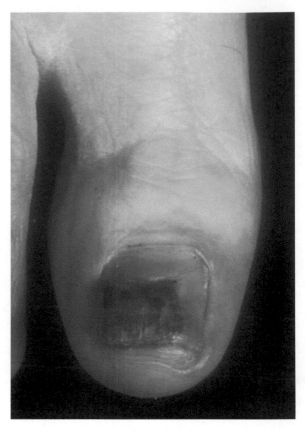

Figure 10.30 Subungual haematoma, sometimes arising from regular minimal trauma. To help distinguish a haematoma from malignant melanoma, the purplish haematoma has a proximal linear edge half way along the great toe nail and the nail-fold itself is not affected.

CHAPTER 11

Non-melanocytic tumours

BENIGN SKIN TUMOURS
Benign epidermal lesions
Benign dermal lesions

LOW-GRADE MALIGNANT SKIN TUMOURS
MALIGNANT SKIN TUMOURS

BENIGN SKIN TUMOURS

Benign epidermal lesions

Common benign epidermal lesions include actinic keratoses, solar lentigos, seborrhoeic keratoses, dermatosis papulosa nigra in black skin, and **skin tags (fibroepithelial polyps)**. Epidermal cysts may be quite large (Chapter 3) or tiny, then usually referred to as milia. Benign melanocytic naevi are derived from melanocytes that reside in the basal layer of the epidermis (Chapter 10).

Actinic keratoses (solar keratoses) are red or light brown, hyperkeratotic lesions which commonly occur on the sun-exposed skin (face, scalp, dorsa of hands) of fair-skinned individuals. There is a small potential for the development of squamous cell carcinoma (about 1 in 1000), and actinic keratoses are sometimes referred to as 'precancers'.

> **Therapeutic suggestions**
> Sunscreens
> Cryotherapy
> Topical 5-fluorouracil
> Topical diclofenac
>
> **Second-line treatment**
> Topical imiquimod

A **seborrhoeic keratosis (basal cell papilloma)** is typically a grey or brown, hyperkeratotic, warty lesion, occurring on the face or trunk, usually in the elderly. Seborrhoeic keratoses are often multiple and are generally easily distinguishable from melanocytic naevi and malignant melanoma.

Rarely, the rapid eruption of multiple pruritic seborrhoeic keratoses on the trunk, particularly when accompanied by acanthosis nigricans, is considered to be associated with an underlying neoplasm. The validity of this Leser–Trélat sign has been questioned by some.

> **Therapeutic suggestions**
> Reassurance
> Curettage and electrodesiccation/'cautery'
>   (C and C)
> Cryotherapy

Dermatosis papulosa nigra comprises a group of small deeply pigmented warty lesions, histologically similar to seborrhoeic keratoses, and commonly occurring on the cheeks of black patients.

Milia are small white epidermal cysts that are frequently seen on the face; they also occur at the site of healed blisters, as seen in the porphyrias and pompholyx. Histiocytomas (dermatofibromas), although dermal in origin (Chapter 6), sometimes produce some epidermal change and are often attached to the overlying epidermis, which can be demonstrated by squeezing the lesion with the fingers.

Facial lesions of similar clinical appearance to clusters of milia have been described in children of West Indian origin, under the acronym of **FACE (facial Afro-Caribbean eruption)**. This is a papular eruption of the face, with numerous lesions around the mouth, eyes, and ears. Pustules are said not to be a feature but there is probably some overlap with children with perioral dermatitis. Spontaneous resolution usually occurs after several months.

Benign dermal lesions

Benign dermal tumours include dermatofibromas, cherry angiomas (Campbell de Morgan spots), and vascular lesions such as strawberry naevi, port-wine stains, and pyogenic granulomas (Chapter 6). Chondrodermatitis nodularis helicis (CNH) is an important painful lesion on the ear which may be mistaken for a basal cell carcinoma (BCC) or a squamous cell carcinoma (SCC). A keratoacanthoma must be distinguished from an SCC.

Chondrodermatitis nodularis helicis presents as a painful nodule on the ear, usually the outer helix in elderly men or the inner helix in elderly women. Regular pressure on the ear when sleeping plays a role in the aetiology but actinic damage seems to be relevant since chondrodermatitis nodularis is more common in fair-skinned individuals who live in sunny climates (e.g. Australasia).

> **Therapeutic suggestions**
> Pressure-relieving material
> Cryotherapy
> Excision of cartilage

A **keratoacanthoma** is characteristically a dome-shaped lesion with a central keratotic plug, growing rapidly (usually developing within about 4 weeks) on sun-exposed skin. Untreated lesions resolve spontaneously over about 6 months, to leave a puckered scar. Keratoacanthomas are generally best excised in order to distinguish histologically from an SCC (which sometimes also grows rapidly) and to yield a better cosmetic result. Keratoacanthomas are sometimes regarded histologically as low-grade malignant lesions but they behave in a benign way clinically.

> **Therapeutic suggestions**
> Excision
> Curettage and electrodesiccation/'cautery'
>   (C and C)
>
> **Second-line treatment**
> Intralesional methotrexate

LOW-GRADE MALIGNANT SKIN TUMOURS

This group includes Bowen's disease (intraepidermal carcinoma, squamous cell carcinoma in situ), arguably keratoacanthoma, and lentigo maligna (Hutchinson's melanotic freckle) (Chapter 10).

Bowen's disease is relatively common in white skin, presenting as red scaly plaques, often on the lower legs. With treatment, the risk of progression to invasive SCC (i.e. with dermal involvement) is about 3%.

> **Therapeutic suggestions**
> Curettage and electrodesiccation/'cautery'
>   (C and C)
> Cryotherapy
> Excision
>
> **Second-line treatment**
> Topical 5-fluorouracil
> Photodynamic therapy
> Topical imiquimod

MALIGNANT SKIN TUMOURS

The role of prolonged sun exposure in the pathogenesis of BCC and SCC, in addition to malignant melanoma, is well recognized. Other predisposing factors for non-melanoma skin cancer (NMSC) include ingested chemicals (e.g. arsenic in medicinal tonics in the past), radiotherapy, chronic scarring (e.g. a burn or traumatic ulcer), immunodeficiency (as seen with immunosuppressed renal transplant patients), and genetic disorders (e.g. xeroderma pigmentosum and the basal cell naevus syndrome). Radiotherapy is a recognized treatment of BCC and SCC but should be reserved for elderly patients because of the risk of further skin cancer in the long term.

Basal cell carcinoma (basal cell epithelioma, BCC) is a relatively common tumour, usually occurring on the head and neck of elderly patients who have had much chronic sun exposure relative to their skin type. A typical slowly growing lesion is a pearly papule with telangiectatic vessels within it. Older lesions may be ulcerated, with a characteristic rolled edge, there being a variable degree of erosion of the underlying tissues (hence the term 'rodent ulcer'). Lesions may be pigmented and on the trunk BCCs are frequently superficial.

Therapeutic suggestions
Excision
Curettage and electrodesiccation/'cautery' (C and C)
Topical imiquimod (superficial BCCs)
Cryotherapy

Second-line treatment
Mohs' micrographic surgery
Radiotherapy

Squamous cell carcinoma (SCC) is generally more aggressive than BCC, with the potential for metastasis to local lymph nodes. Irregular keratotic, ulcerated tumours usually take a few months to develop (helping to distinguish from a keratoacanthoma), the head and neck being the most frequently affected sites. Squamous carcinomas may be more aggressive at certain sites, including the ear and the lip. An SCC sometimes arises in chronically ulcerated skin (Marjolin's ulcer).

Therapeutic suggestions
Wide excision

Second-line treatment
Mohs' micrographic surgery
Radiotherapy

Epithelial tumours are rare in black skin, unless there is an underlying pigmentary disorder such as albinism.

Uncommon tumours of the epidermis include **Paget's disease of the nipple** and **extramammary Paget's disease**, usually affecting the perianal and genital regions. The occurrence of dermal tumours, particularly on the scalp, should always raise the suspicion of **skin metastases** from a primary tumour elsewhere (e.g. breast, lung, or kidney). The lesions of various types of **cutaneous T-cell lymphoma** (including mycosis fungoides) and **B-cell lymphoma** are also predominantly dermal (Chapter 6).

FURTHER READING

Bolognia JL, Jorrizzo JL, Rapini RP, et al (eds). Dermatology. Philadelphia: Mosby, 2003.

Burns T, Breathnach S, Cox N, Griffiths C (eds). Rook's Textbook of Dermatology, 7th edn. Oxford: Blackwell Science, 2004.

Gawkrodger DJ. Dermatology: An Illustrated Colour Text, 3rd edn. Edinburgh: Churchill Livingstone, 2002.

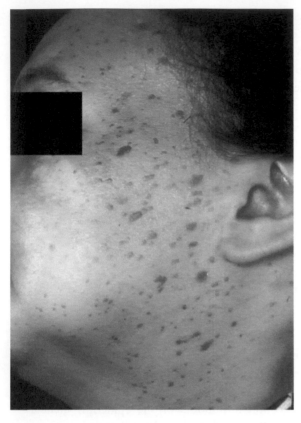

Figure 11.1   Numerous darkly pigmented seborrhoeic keratoses on the cheek of a black woman.

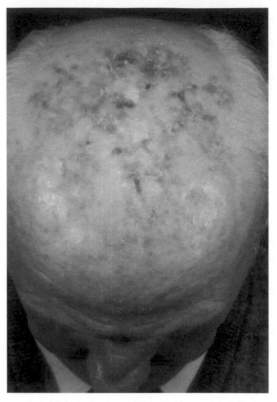

Figure 11.3   Actinic (solar) keratosis, with multiple keratoses on the bald scalp of a man with a Celtic (fair-skinned) complexion and extensive sun damage.

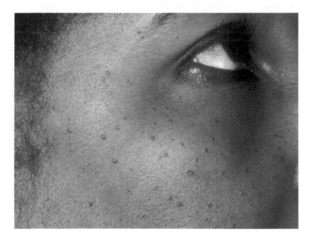

Figure 11.2   Dermatosis papulosa nigra, showing multiple tiny black warty lesions on the cheek of a woman of Afro-Caribbean origin. The histology is similar to that of a seborrhoeic keratosis. Dermatosis papulosa nigra is commonly seen in black people.

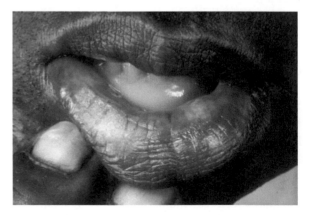

Figure 11.4   Leucokeratosis, showing white hyperkeratotic lesions on the lower lip of a black man. These changes are usually considered to represent solar keratoses on the lip.

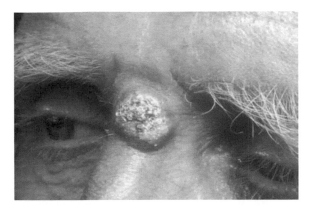

Figure 11.5 Keratoacanthoma, showing a solitary dome-shaped lesion on the bridge of the nose. The lesion had developed rapidly (within 4 weeks) and the characteristic central plug can be seen.

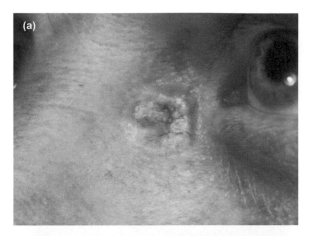

(a)

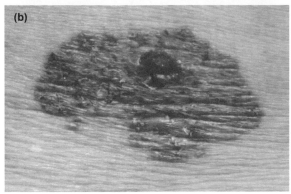

(b)

Figure 11.7a and b Basal cell carcinoma (basal cell epithelioma). (11.7a) A typical pearly lesion with a rolled edge and prominent telangiectatic vessels adjacent to the right inner canthus. (11.7b) A larger pigmented superficial basal cell carcinoma on the upper back.

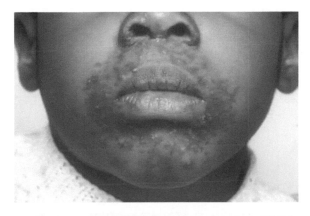

Figure 11.6 Facial Afro-Caribbean eruption (FACE), showing lesions resembling milia in the perioral region of a young boy of Afro-Caribbean origin, in whom there was thought to be a degree of perioral dermatitis. This disorder tends to eventually resolve spontaneously. The papular lesions commonly affect the forehead and are usually accompanied by post-inflammatory hyperpigmentation.

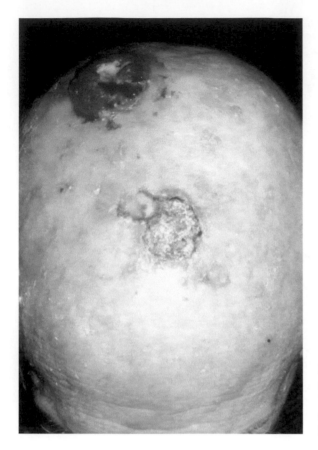

Figure 11.8   Squamous cell carcinoma, showing a large circular fleshy tumour on the posterior vertex of a bald scalp. The irregular keratotic lesion on the anterior scalp was also a squamous cell carcinoma and there are numerous actinic keratoses.

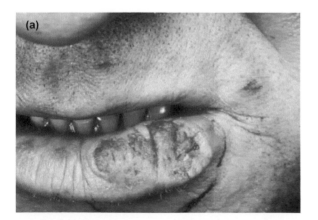

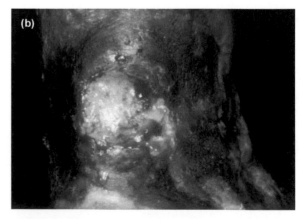

Figure 11.9a and b   Squamous cell carcinoma, with an irregular slow-growing keratotic and crusted lesion on the lower lip (11.9a), the site of excessive sun exposure over the years. A long-standing leg ulcer rarely develops into a squamous carcinoma (Marjolin's ulcer) (11.9b).

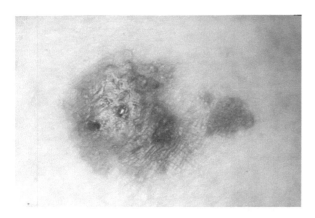

Figure 11.10   Bowen's disease (intraepidermal carcinoma, squamous cell carcinoma in situ), showing a reddish-brown scaly plaque on the lower leg. Other common sites for Bowen's disease include the face and dorsa of hands.

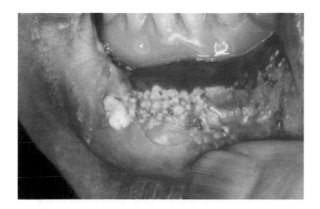

Figure 11.11   Leukoplakia, affecting the mucosal surface of the lower lip. This premalignant disorder should be distinguished from other examples of white mucosal patches, including candida and lichen sclerosus et atrophicus, the latter tending to affect the genital

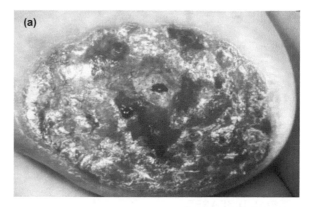

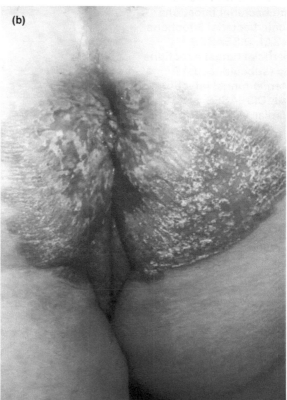

Figure 11.12a and b   Paget's disease. (11.12a) Paget's disease of the nipple, associated with an undorlying intraductal carcinoma of the breast. The similarity to extramammary Paget's disease, in this case affecting the perianal region (11.12b) is readily apparent.

CHAPTER 12

Infectious diseases and infestations

BACTERIAL DISEASES
Acute bacterial infections
Chronic bacterial infections
FUNGAL DISEASES
Superficial fungal infections
Deep (subcutaneous) fungal infections
Systemic fungal infections
VIRAL DISEASES
Vesicular viral infections

Viral exanthems
Viral warts
HIV and Kaposi's sarcoma
COMMON PARASITIC DISEASES
INFESTATIONS
Scabies
Insect bites
Lice infestations

BACTERIAL DISEASES

Bacterial infections of the skin usually develop as a result of previous damage to the skin by a physical agent or disease process (e.g. atopic dermatitis), which allows a portal of entry for the microorganism. Most infections are due to organisms which are not normally part of the resident flora, particularly *Streptococcus pyogenes* (group A streptococcus) and *Staphylococcus aureus*, the clinical features of the infection depending on the depth of skin inflammation.

Acute bacterial infections

Erysipelas is a streptococcal infection, involving the superficial lymphatic vessels, which usually follows a minor abrasion. Typically there is a red oedematous area of skin, often on the lower leg or cheek, with a sharply demarcated border, accompanied by pyrexia and leukocytosis. **Cellulitis** is usually a streptococcal infection, involving the deeper layers of the skin, although the distinction between erysipelas and cellulitis is of little clinical importance. A red hot tender area of skin (e.g. surrounding a leg ulcer) is generally accompanied by pyrexia, leukocytosis, and lymphadenopathy.

> **Therapeutic suggestions**
> Intravenous benzyl penicillin and flucloxacillin
> Oral penicillin V and flucloxacillin
>
> **Second-line treatment**
> Oral ciprofloxacin

Impetigo is a superficial skin infection usually due to *Streptococcus pyogenes* and/or *Staphylococcus aureus*. Red, vesicular, or pustular lesions develop into golden crusts. Bullous impetigo is due to a toxin released from *Staphylococcus aureus*.

> **Therapeutic suggestions**
> Topical antibiotics
> Oral antibiotics

As in impetigo, **ecthyma** is caused by *Streptococcus pyogenes* and/or *Staphylococcus aureus*, but the infection occurs at a deeper level in the skin. Ecthyma is often seen in patients with poor hygiene and nutritional status, beginning with vesicles or bullae, which break down to form crusts, which, in turn, commonly ulcerate.

Infection of a hair follicle with *Staphylococcus aureus* produces a **furuncle (boil)**, whereas a **carbuncle** affects several adjacent hair follicles, discharging pus through multiple sinuses. **Folliculitis**, or inflammation of the opening of hair follicles, may be caused by bacteria or fungi. Commonly, no infective organism is isolated. The problems encountered by black patients with **pseudofolliculitis** of the beard area have been discussed in Chapter 3.

Less common bacterial infections include erythrasma, caused by *Corynebacterium minutissimum*, erysipeloid, caused by *Erysipelothrix rhusiopathiae*, and **anthrax**, caused by *Bacillus anthracis*.

Erythrasma consists of reddish-brown, slightly scaly, confluent lesions in the groins or axillae, the lesions fluorescing with Wood's light to produce a coral red colour (Chapter 1).

Therapeutic suggestions
Topical miconazole
Topical clotrimazole
Topical econazole
Oral erythromycin

Second-line treatment
Clarithromycin

Occasionally, *Streptococcus pyogenes* alone or sometimes multiple organisms acting synergistically will produce a **necrotizing fasciitis**, in which the treatment of choice is early surgical debridement in addition to appropriate antibiotic therapy. Bacterial synergistic gangrene may run a particularly fulminant course in patients with diabetes mellitus or poor nutritional status.

Chronic bacterial infections

Syphilis, caused by the spirochaete *Treponema pallidum*, is relatively common and the skin may be affected in the primary, secondary, or tertiary stages. An indurated painless chancre usually occurs as a single lesion on the penis or vulva (where it may not be noticed) but other sites may be involved. The eruption of secondary syphilis is variable but a papulosquamous rash is frequently seen on the trunk and limbs, lesions on the palms and soles providing a stong clue to the diagnosis. At this stage the patient may have malaise with a headache, low-grade fever, generalized lymphadenopathy, mucosal lesions, patchy alopecia, and condyloma lata, which are particularly infectious. In tertiary syphilis, there may be a solitary, chronic, indurated plaque or group of nodules.

Lyme disease (erythema chronicum migrans) is caused by the spirochaete *Borrelia burgdorferi* following a tick bite. The initial lesion is a red macule, which slowly enlarges to form an annular plaque. Secondary lesions, including blotchy erythema or urticaria, may develop, accompanied by signs of systemic upset and lymphadenopathy.

Tuberculosis of the skin may be localized or disseminated, the type of lesion depending on whether there is primary inoculation of a non-immune host or skin involvement via lymphatic or haematogenous spread in a patient with evidence of tuberculosis elsewhere.

In developed countries, cutaneous tuberculosis is uncommon but is more common in immigrants (e.g. from Asia). A number of patterns have been described. In a non-immune host, a **tuberculous chancre** presents as an inflammatory nodule accompanied by lymphadenitis and regional lymphadenopathy. In previously exposed hosts the lesions may take the form of verrucous nodules (**tuberculosis verrucosa**) or the chronic scarring process of **lupus vulgaris**, often seen on the face. In **scrofuloderma**, tuberculous lymph nodes or bone forms a fistula with the overlying skin. The term **papulonecrotic tuberculid** is applied to a symmetrical papular eruption of the face and limbs, each lesion undergoing central necrosis and scarring. **Miliary tuberculosis**, caused by haematogenous spread in patients with fulminant tuberculosis, is rare.

Therapeutic suggestions
Antituberculous drugs

Fish tank granuloma (swimming pool granuloma) is caused by *Mycobacterium marinum* and particularly occurs in the handlers of sick tropical fish or sometimes in children as a result of swimming in pools where the organism is prevalent. Minor trauma usually precedes the development of a circular reddish-brown nodule or plaque on the dorsum of the hand and proximal lesions may ensue by 'sporotrichoid spread', in which lesions occur along the distribution of the lymphatics.

Therapeutic suggestions
Minocycline
Co-trimoxazole

Second-line treatment
Rifampicin

Leprosy is endemic in many parts of the world. There is a spectrum of disease, depending on the ability of the host to mount an immune response to the *Mycobacterium leprae*. In **tuberculoid leprosy**, few or no bacilli are seen in typically macular hypopigmented anaesthetic lesions, but there may be severe disability as a result of immunologically mediated neurological damage. At the other end of the spectrum, the characteristic lesions of **lepromatous leprosy** are nodules on the earlobes, face, trunk, and extremities, each lesion containing numerous bacilli. **Borderline leprosy** is subclassified into borderline tuberculoid (BT) and borderline lepromatous (BL) forms, and the precise type may vary in an individual.

Therapeutic suggestions
Rifampicin
Dapsone
Clofazimine

Second-line treatment
Minocycline
Clarithromycin

Yaws and **pinta** are both treponemal infections and, as in syphilis, there are primary and chronic skin manifestations. The aetiology of **tropical ulcer** is a little uncertain, the role of the spirochaete mouth commensal *Borrelia vincentii* being disputed. Typically, a haemorrhagic papule at the site of trauma breaks down to form a slough-based, sharply defined necrotic ulcer, particularly on the lower leg (Chapter 7).

FUNGAL DISEASES

Fungal infections of the skin may be considered as superficial, deep (subcutaneous), and systemic infections. Superficial infections are common in most countries, whereas deep and systemic fungal infections tend to be confined to tropical and subtropical countries.

Superficial fungal infections

Dermatophyte infections can affect various regions of the body, the fungi colonizing keratinized tissue such as stratum corneum, nails, and hair. The three genera of dermatophytes are *Trichophyton*, *Microsporum*, and *Epidermophyton*.

Athlete's foot (tinea pedis) usually presents with sore, itchy, moist white fissures in the toe webs but may be more extensive. **Tinea corporis**, commonly due to *Trichophyton rubrum*, comprises reddish scaly plaques with an active red advancing edge and central clearing. It is often unilateral, at least to begin with.

Therapeutic suggestions
Topical terbinafine
Topical clotrimazole

The nails of **tinea unguium** are thickened, discoloured, and powdery in appearance, the process usually beginning distally and moving proximally. The organisms most frequently isolated are *Trichophyton rubrum*, *Trichophyton interdigitale*, and *Epidermophyton floccosum*.

Therapeutic suggestions
Oral terbinafine
Itraconazole

Second-line treatment
Topical amorolfine

Scalp ringworm (tinea capitis) may be caused by *Trichophyton tonsurans*, *Microsporum canis*, *Trichophyton rubrum*, or *Trichophyton verrucosum*. There is inflammation, hair loss, and scarring. Infection of the hair shaft with *Trichophyton verrucosum* may cause a pronounced inflammatory reaction or **kerion**. At present, scalp ringworm is very common in Afro-Caribbean schoolchildren in the UK and elsewhere in the world, the usual organism being *Trichophyton tonsurans*.

Therapeutic suggestions
Griseofulvin
Oral terbinafine
Itraconazole

Napkin candidiasis and **candidal intertrigo** (affecting the skin folds) are caused by *Candida albicans*, often complicating an irritant dermatitis. Characteristically there are red shiny patches, with 'satellite' lesions. Candidal paronychia, a hazard of regular immersion of the hands in water, presents with a boggy inflamed nail fold, accompanied by pus.

Therapeutic suggestions
Topical antifungals
Topical antifungal/corticosteroid combination

Second-line treatment
Oral antifungals

In black patients, the erythematous inflammatory reaction to superficial fungal infections is often absent and the diagnosis is based on the characteristic shape and the distribution of the epidermal lesions, preferably confirmed by positive mycology in skin scrapings (or nail clippings for tinea unguium). Hair pullings and/or hair brushings are used to confirm a diagnosis of tinea capitis.

Pityriasis versicolor (tinea versicolor), caused by *Malassezia furfur*, is common, particularly in young adults. In a white patient without a suntan, there are usually pink circular or oval, coalescing lesions on the trunk, upper arms, and neck, with fine scaling. Patients often present with pityriasis versicolor after a sunbathing holiday, and it is common to see slightly scaly, hypopigmented, coalescing lesions. The distribution of the lesions and hypopigmentation rather than depigmentation helps to distinguish pityriasis versicolor from vitiligo. In black skin, hypopigmentation or sometimes hyperpigmentation may be seen in a typical distribution (Chapter 1).

The hypopigmentation associated with pityriasis versicolor is thought to be due to the inhibition of tyrosinase in melanocytes by azelaic acid, produced by the conversion of fatty acids in the skin by yeast enzymes.

Therapeutic suggestions
Topical clotrimazole
Topical ketoconazole
Topical terbinafine

Second-line treatment
Itraconazole

Deep (subcutaneous) fungal infections

Sporotrichosis, caused by *Sporothrix schenckii*, usually presents as a chronic infection with nodules that drain and suppurate, often slowly progressing proximally along the distribution of the lymphatics.

Therapeutic suggestions
Potassium iodide
Oral terbinafine

Second-line treatment
Itraconazole

In **chromoblastomycosis (chromomycosis)**, one usually sees verrucous nodules and plaques on the lower legs and feet, typically in farmers from tropical and subtropical areas. Pink scaly plaques subsequently become verrucous with characteristic 'black dots' on the surface, due to transepidermal elimination of fungi and dermal constituents.

Mycetoma is a localized, chronic infection with various species of fungi or actinomycetes, resulting in severe damage to the skin, subcutaneous tissues, and often the bones of the feet or hands. Granules are produced within granulomas and abscesses, and are discharged to the surface through draining sinuses.

Systemic fungal infections

These include **coccidioidomycosis**, caused by *Coccidioides immitis*, **blastomycosis**, caused by *Blastomyces dermatitidis*, **histoplasmosis**, caused by *Histoplasma capsulatum*, and the opportunistic systemic mycoses, **cryptococcus**, caused by *Cryptococcus neoformans*, and **aspergillosis**, the skin lesions usually being caused by *Aspergillus flavus*. The primary airborne infection may be limited to the lungs, cutaneous involvement resulting from systemic spread of these fungi.

Investigation of bacterial and fungal diseases
Swabs
Skin scrapings and strippings
Nail and subungual samples
Hair pullings and hairbrush samples
Pus aspirates and biopsies
Blood cultures

VIRAL DISEASES

Vesicular viral infections

Herpes simplex virus (HSV) infections are seen in a number of clinical situations, including herpes labialis ('cold sores'), herpetic whitlow (on the fingertip), eczema herpeticum (a potentially serious complication of atopic dermatitis, Chapter 2), and genital herpes. HSV-1 is most often associated with lesions on the lips and HSV-2 with genital lesions, although this may vary. Typically, a painful cluster of vesicles on an erythematous base becomes crusted, before resolving spontaneously after a few days.

Therapeutic suggestions
Topical aciclovir
Oral aciclovir
Sunscreens

Herpes zoster (shingles) is caused by herpes virus varicellae (the reactivated chickenpox virus). Dermatomal pain is followed by a linear, red, macular, papular, vesicular, then pustular eruption. Post-herpetic neuralgia (persistent pain) occurs in about 10% of patients, being more common and severe in the elderly.

Therapeutic suggestions
Oral aciclovir
Oral famciclovir
Oral valaciclovir

Chickenpox (varicella) and **hand-foot-and-mouth disease**, usually caused by a Coxsackie virus, are common infections in children. Human **orf** is a contagious vesicular disease caused by paravaccinia virus (a pox virus), contracted from direct contact with infected sheep and goats.

Viral exanthems

Viral exanthems (e.g. measles, roseola, rubella) commonly present to the family practitioner. **Erythema infectiosum (fifth disease)**, caused by a parvovirus, has a characteristic rash with the 'slapped cheek' appearance, with perioral pallor. Unlike in measles, there is little or no prodromal illness. After 1–2 days, the rash on the cheeks fades, the characteristic reticulate eruption on the limbs and upper trunk occurring after 1–4 days, before gradually fading.

Viral warts

Warts or verrucae are very common, resulting from infection of epithelial cells by human papillomavirus (HPV). The appearance of the wart depends on the site involved, the type of infecting papillomavirus, and the immunological response of the host. Clinical variants include common warts (e.g. on the hands), **plane warts** (often on the face), **plantar warts** (commonly termed **verrucae**), and genital warts.

Therapeutic suggestions
Salicylic acid preparations
Cryotherapy
Adhesive (duct) tape

Genital warts may be small individual lesions or may coalesce into large cauliflower-like 'condyloma acuminata'. Colposcopy for female genital warts and proctoscopy for homosexual males may be required to identify and treat any cervical or rectal warts because of the risk of malignant change. Sexual partners should also be examined.

Therapeutic suggestions
Topical imiquimod
Topical podophyllotoxin
Cryotherapy

Bowenoid papulosis is a multicentric disorder caused by a human papillomavirus infection. It usually presents with reddish papules and plaques on the penis, vulva, or perianal region, and this intraepidermal dysplastic disease should be distinguished from Bowen's disease, since extensive surgery is not indicated for Bowenoid papulosis.

Epidermodysplasia verruciformis is a rare clinical entity in which multiple plane warts develop in sheets, sometimes affecting much of the skin. The warts usually occur in childhood but can begin later in life. Resistance to treatment is common and there is a risk of the development of squamous cell carcinoma, particularly on sun exposed sites.

The lesions of **molluscum contagiosum**, caused by a pox virus, comprise reddish papules, each often having an umbilicated centre. They are usually multiple, commonly occurring on the trunk or proximal limbs of children, and resolve spontaneously.

Investigation of viral diseases
Electron microscopy of vesicle fluid
Viral culture (e.g. HSV)
Antigen detection (using PCR)
Tzanck smear*
Serological antibody detection

*A **Tzanck smear** (as outlined in Chapter 5) is still useful in confirming herpes infection. Bullae should be new and not infected with bacteria. The roof is removed and the floor scraped with a scalpel. The sample is then spread onto a glass slide, air-dried or fixed by immersion 4–5 times in 95% ethyl alcohol. The best stain is Giemsa, which requires only 2–3 minutes. Microscopic examination can be immediate. In herpes, multinucleate giant cells and inclusion bodies are seen.

HIV and Kaposi's sarcoma

Acute primary human immunodeficiency virus (HIV) infection is often asymptomatic but symptoms of variable severity occur in about 50% of patients. Following an incubation period of 14 days, there may be fever, malaise, headache, sore throat, lymphadenopathy, arthralgia, abdominal pain, and diarrhoea. An asymptomatic maculopapular rash occurs about 1 week later and settles within 1–3 days. Urticaria, palatal erythema, and palatal erosions may occur. The illness resolves usually within 2 weeks, a more prolonged course sometimes being associated with a poor prognosis.

During the acute illness, HIV can be cultured from peripheral blood lymphocytes and p24 antigen detected. Seroconversion often occurs within 4–6 weeks of the acute illness but HIV antibodies may not be detected until a period of 6 months. Seroconversion illness is diagnosed by positive plasma HIV polymerase chain reaction (PCR), accompanied by negative or equivocal HIV antibody tests.

The incidence of Kaposi's sarcoma (KS) in acquired immunodeficiency syndrome (AIDS) is about 40% in homosexual males, occurring in only 5% of other groups with AIDS, e.g. haemophiliacs,

renal transplant recipients, and Africans. As discussed in Chapter 6, there is good evidence that the herpes virus HHV8 is the cause of KS, whether seen in association with HIV infection or not. This virus is sometimes referred to as the Kaposi's sarcoma herpes virus (KSHV).

In most cases, the course of Kaposi's sarcoma in AIDS is insidious but it occasionally behaves aggressively, death usually resulting from lung involvement. In the skin there are reddish-purple or brown coloured dermal lesions which can be macules, nodules, or plaques. These are sometimes arranged in the skin creases (e.g. on the trunk) or at the site of trauma. Common sites include the tip of the nose, lips, the trunk, and mucosal surfaces including the hard palate and tongue.

Other skin manifestations of AIDS include worsening of seborrhoeic dermatitis or psoriasis, seborrhoeic folliculitis, herpes zoster, herpes simplex, candidiasis, dermatophyte infections, molluscum contagiosum warts, and drug eruptions. Oral hairy leukoplakia usually affects the lateral border of the tongue and is caused by the Epstein–Barr virus, which can also cause lymphomas in AIDS.

COMMON PARASITIC DISEASES

Cutaneous larva migrans (creeping eruption) is a parasitic infection caused by the larvae of animal intestinal hookworms (e.g. *Ankylostoma brasiliensis*) burrowing into the skin, after contact with the beach or soil. A red itchy papule is followed by the development of migrating serpiginous channels, reflecting movement of the larvae within the epidermis and upper dermis.

Therapeutic suggestions
Topical thiabendazole
Oral albendazole

Onchocerciasis is extremely common in certain tropical areas of the world, being caused by the nematode *Onchocerca volvulus*, which is transmitted to human skin in larval form by black fly or gnat bites. Patients develop itching followed by excoriations, lichenification, pigmentary changes, and lymphadenopathy. Subcutaneous infestation with the adult worms leads to oedema, nodules, and sometimes large asymptomatic tumours. Increased pigmentation commonly accompanies lichenification of the back and buttocks. Onchocercal depigmentation occurs in long-standing onchodermatitis in African skin, often accompanied by fixed inguinal lymphadenopathy.

> **Therapeutic suggestions**
> Ivermectin
>
> **Second-line treatment**
> Oral albendazole

Leishmaniasis is a protozoan infection, transmitted by sandfly bites, which occurs as three predominant clinical forms: cutaneous leishmaniasis (Oriental sore), caused by *Leishmania tropica*; American cutaneous and mucocutaneous leishmaniasis, caused by *Leishmania braziliensis*; and visceral leishmaniasis (kala-azar), caused by *Leishmania donovani*. Bites on the face, arms, and hands progress to ulcerating nodules, which discharge and crust over. The natural history, in the absence of treatment, is to eventually heal with unsightly cribriform scarring. Some patients with visceral leishmaniasis develop reddish and/or hypopigmented nodular lesions, referred to as post-kala-azar dermal leishmaniasis.

> **Therapeutic suggestions**
> Pentavalent antimonials
>
> **Second-line treatment**
> Rifampicin
> Cryotherapy

Other parasitic skin diseases include myiasis (caused by the larvae of dipterous flies), schistosomiasis (caused by trematode flukes), cercarial dermatitis (swimmer's itch), and amoebic abscesses.

INFESTATIONS

Infestation may be defined as the harbouring of insect or worm parasites in or on the body. In temperate climates insect life on the skin is usually short-lived. Common problems include scabies, insect bites, and various forms of lice infestation, especially head lice.

Scabies

Scabies is caused by the scabies mite, *Sarcoptes scabiei*, symptoms occurring when the host develops an allergic reaction to the female mite. Patients usually complain of an extremely itchy, red, papular rash, particularly affecting the finger webs, hands, wrists, and pubic area. The mite can be extracted from a linear burrow using various techniques, as described in Chapter 1. Affected individuals may be asymptomatic and all occupants and regular visitors to the home should be treated.

> **Therapeutic suggestions**
> Permethrin 5% cream
> Malathion 5% lotion
>
> **Second-line treatment**
> Ivermectin

Insect bites

Insect bites often occur on covered skin, and frequently encountered beasts include fleas and bed bugs. Individual lesions comprise reddish papules, sometimes with a central punctum, and surrounding erythema. Characteristically, the lesions occur in a linear pattern and they are sometimes blistered. Insect bite reactions may persist for several weeks.

Mosquito and gnat bites are common, the reaction of individuals being rather variable. Some people are bitten more frequently than others, and some react much more than others. Caterpillar bites often become eczematized, justifying the clinical description of caterpillar dermatitis. Exogenous lesions may also be inflicted by spiders, ants, ticks, chiggers (harvest mites), blister beetles, and kissing bugs. Spider bites are often necrotic in the centre of the lesions.

Lice infestations

Lice are responsible for the diseases **pediculosis capitis** (caused by the head louse), **pediculosis corporis** (caused by the body louse), and **pediculosis pubis** (caused by the pubic louse).

Many children, particularly those attending school, have nits (head louse eggs) attached to scalp hair, sometimes with excoriation and secondary infection. Recurrent infestation with head lice is common, despite good personal hygiene.

Pediculosis corporis usually occurs in individuals with poor personal hygiene, presenting with itching, excoriation, and secondary infection. Lice are rarely seen on the skin and it is important to examine the seams of clothing in order to confirm the diagnosis. Pediculosis pubis presents with suprapubic itching and the appearance of 'black dots' in the pubic hair.

FURTHER READING

Bolognia JL, Jorrizzo JL, Rapini RP, et al (eds). Dermatology. Philadelphia: Mosby, 2003.

Burns T, Breathnach S, Cox N, Griffiths C (eds). Rook's Textbook of Dermatology, 7th edn. Oxford: Blackwell Science, 2004.

Gawkrodger DJ. Dermatology: An Illustrated Colour Text, 3rd edn. Edinburgh: Churchill Livingstone, 2002.

Glaser DA, Penneys NS. Tests for viral, HIV-related and tropical skin infections. In: Cerio R, Archer CB (eds). Clinical Investigation of Skin Disorders. London: Chapman and Hall Medical, 1998.

Leeming JP, Johnson EM, Warnock DW. Bacteriology and mycology. In: Cerio R, Archer CB (eds). Clinical Investigation of Skin Disorders. London: Chapman and Hall Medical, 1998.

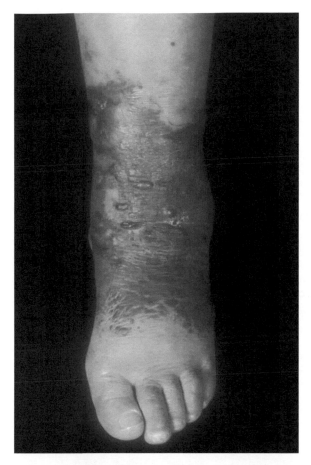

Figure 12.1 Erysipelas, showing a purplish clearly defined painful area on the lower leg and dorsum of the foot.

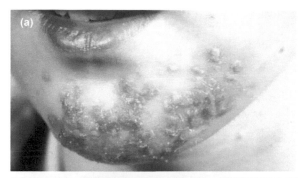

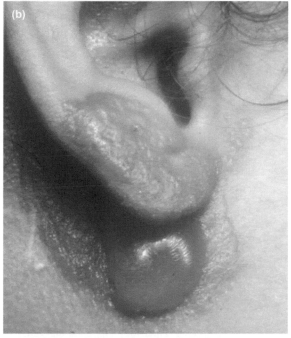

Figure 12.3a and b Impetigo, with golden crusts on the chin (12.3a) and a red inflammatory lesion on the right ear, accompanied by a staphylococcal toxin-induced blister (12.3b). Impetigo, along with insect bite reactions, is a relatively common cause of blistering in childhood.

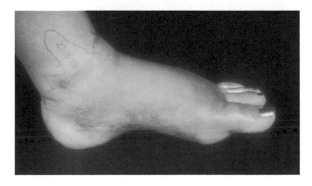

Figure 12.2 Cellulitis, showing a painful diffuse red area of cellulitis on the foot. In erysipelas superficial involvement of the lymphatics characteristically produces an elevated well-demarcated border, whereas cellulitis is a deeper, more diffuse process.

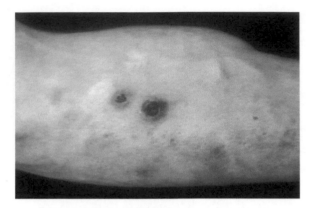

Figure 12.4 Ecthyma, showing numerous red painful lesions in the inframammary region. Ecthyma is a deeper infection than impetigo, usually occurring in patients with poor personal hygiene and nutritional status. Lesions often develop a necrotic centre.

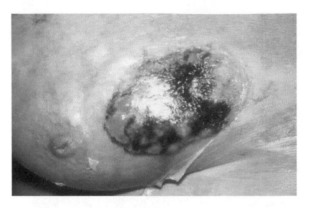

Figure 12.6 Necrotizing fasciitis, in this case an example of fatal bacterial synergistic gangrene in a young woman with diabetes mellitus. The necrotic areas on the breasts betray the depth of the infectious process and, as with a severe cellulitis, blistering of the skin can occur. Necrotizing fasciitis is usually caused by *Streptococcus pyogenes* and early surgical debridement is essential.

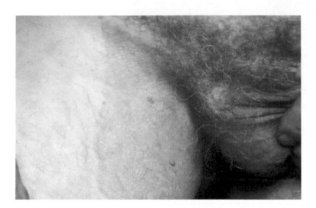

Figure 12.5 Erythrasma, showing a characteristic reddish-brown, slightly scaly confluent area in the groin region of a white man. In deeply pigmented skin the patches are hyperpigmented and examination with Wood's light shows coral red fluorescence (Chapter 1).

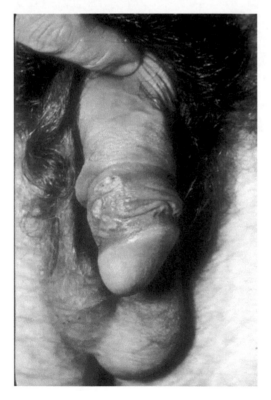

Figure 12.7 Syphilis, showing the primary lesion, a painless chancre, on the penis of a white man. A chancre usually heals in a few weeks to form an atrophic scar, and a chancre affecting the female genitalia may pass unnoticed by the patient. Other sites include the mouth and perianal region.

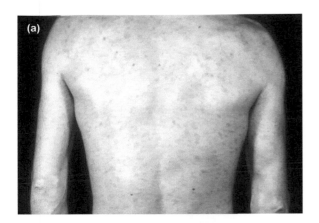

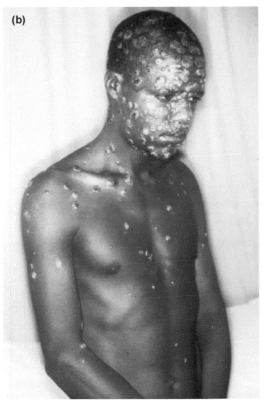

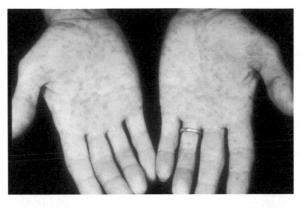

Figure 12.9 Secondary syphilis, showing distinctive red-brown papules on the palms. At this stage there may also be condyloma lata lesions in the perianal region.

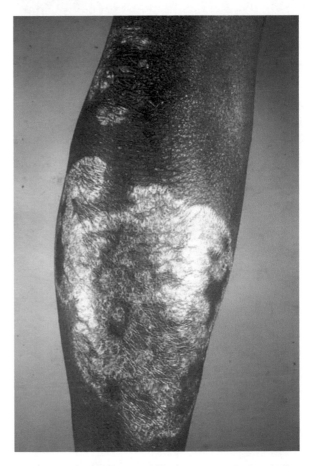

Figure 12.8a and b Secondary syphilis, showing a characteristic symmetrical reddish maculopapular rash on the trunk and arms of a white man (12.8a). This eruption usually appears 8–12 weeks after the primary lesion and may be accompanied by malaise, lymphadenopathy, and mucosal erosions in the oral cavity (snail-track ulcers). 12.8b shows numerous crusted lesions on the face, scalp, trunk, and arms of an African man. Serological tests for syphilis were positive and these unusual lesions rapidly resolved after treatment with penicillin.

Figure 12.10 Tertiary syphilis, less common than in the past, showing silver-grey hyperkeratotic plaques on the arm of a patient with black skin.

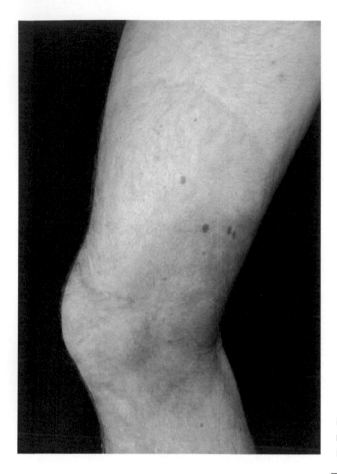

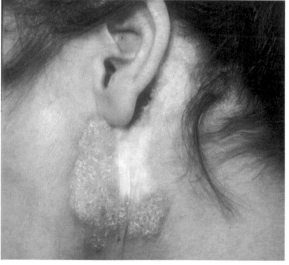

Figure 12.11 Lyme disease (erythema chronicum migrans), showing a tic bite with a surrounding expanding red annular plaque on the arm.

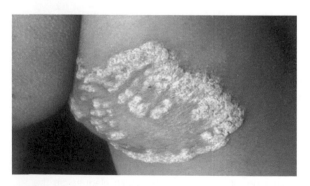

Figure 12.12 Tuberculosis, showing a hyperkeratotic, 'verrucous' plaque on the right buttock of a man with black skin.

Figure 12.13 Tuberculosis, showing the clinical variant lupus vulgaris, with a granulomatous red plaque inferior to the left ear of an Indian woman. Hypopigmented scar tissue is visible posteriorly.

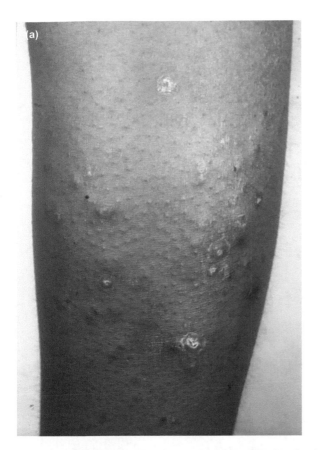

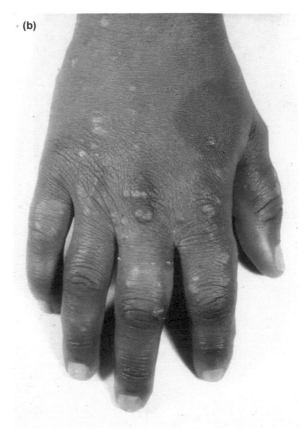

Figure 12.14a and b   Papulonecrotic tuberculid, showing hyperpigmented, hyperkeratotic papules and nodules on the forearm (12.14a) and dorsum of the hand of a black patient (12.14b). This eruption is symmetrical and also affects the face.

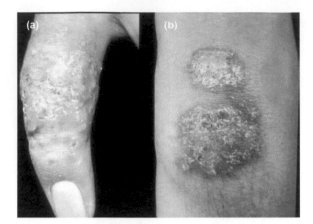

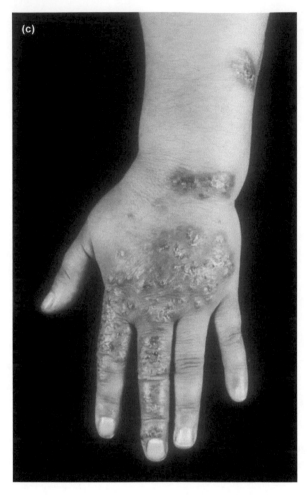

Figure 12.15a, b, and c   Fish tank granuloma, caused by *Mycobacterium marinum*, showing reddish granulomatous plaques on the dorsum of the left index finger (12.15a) and two plaques in the elbow region (12.15b). The lesions are predominantly dermal but there is often an epidermal component, as shown by the scaling. (12.15c) Typical sporotrichoid spread on the hand and forearm of a woman from the Middle East.

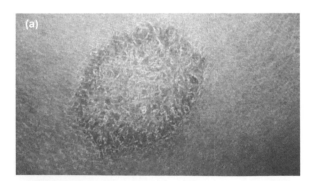

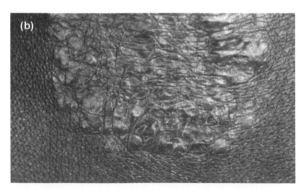

Figure 12.16a and b   Leprosy, showing the clinical variant borderline leprosy. In 12.16a there is a slightly scaly circular plaque, with a hyperpigmented edge in an African man. 12.16b shows subtle wrinkling of a palpable dermal plaque. There may be a few lesions in borderline leprosy, whereas in tuberculoid leprosy there is usually a solitary anaesthetic plaque.

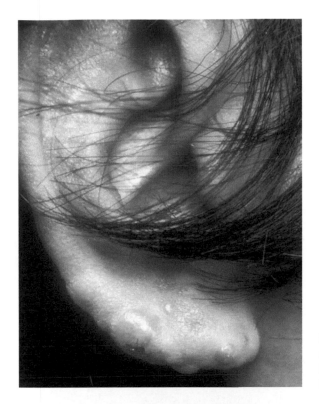

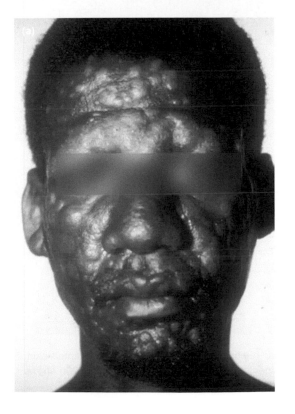

Figure 12.17 Lepromatous leprosy, showing papules and nodules on the earlobe of a man of Indian origin. He also had dermal plaques on the forehead, producing the so-called 'leonine facies'.

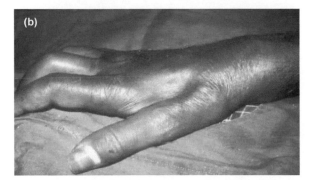

Figure 12.18a and b Leprosy, showing numerous light brown nodules of lepromatous leprosy on the face of an African man (12.18a). Neurological damage is more common at the tuberculoid end of the spectrum, and 12.18b shows the dorsum of the right hand of a woman with deeply pigmented skin with median nerve palsy.

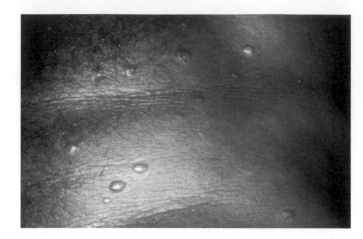

Figure 12.19 Leprosy, showing a number of small brown skin-coloured papules of lepromatous leprosy on the nape of the neck of an African man.

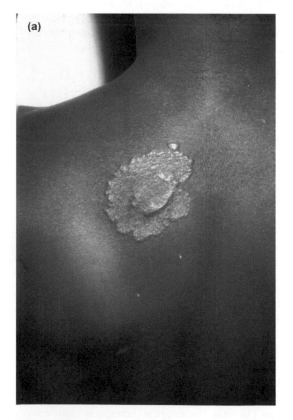

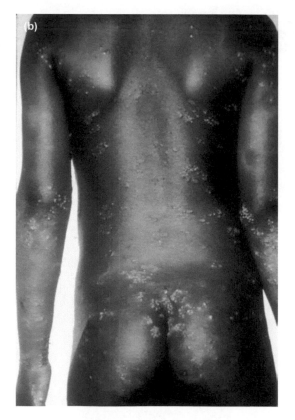

Figure 12.20a and b   Yaws, showing a plaque on the left scapular region of a man with deeply pigmented skin. Note the raised hyperkeratotic centre of the plaque and the hypopigmented surrounding skin (12.20a). 12.20b shows numerous hypopigmented hyperkeratotic lesions on the back, buttocks, and arms.

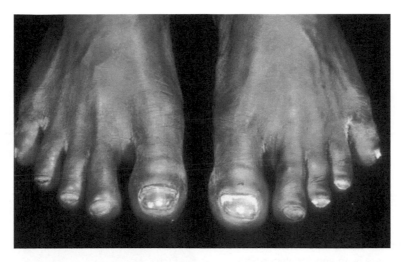

Figure 12.21   Tinea pedis, showing scaly areas on the dorsa of the feet and in the toe webs. In black skin one often sees hyperpigmentation. Tinea pedis is frequently unilateral and may be accompanied by tinea unguium.

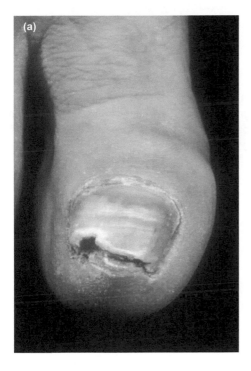

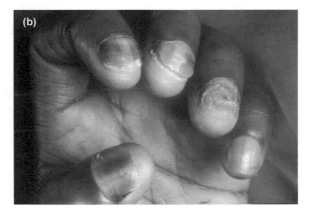

Figure 12.22a and b   Tinea unguium, with prominent nail dystrophy of the great toe nail (12.22a) and finger nails (12.22b). 12.22a shows a characteristic thickened powdery yellowish nail, the pathology beginning distally. In deeply pigmented skin the nail discoloration is more likely to be black (12.22b) or grey. Confirmation of the diagnosis can be made by taking nail clippings and subungual debris for mycology, including microscopy and culture.

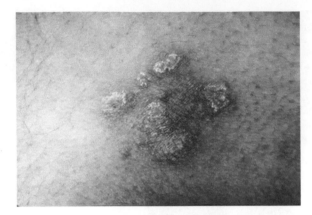

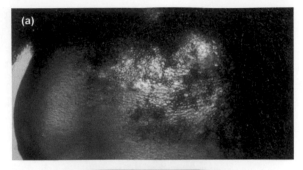

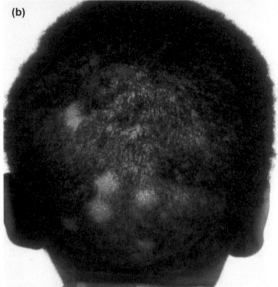

Figure 12.23 Tinea corporis, showing inflammatory scaly lesions on the trunk, caused by *Trichophyton rubrum*. Characteristically there is an annular plaque with central clearing, and an advancing red inflamed border, scrapings from which usually yield positive mycology. In black skin, ringworm is usually accompanied by a degree of post-inflammatory hyperpigmentation. The marked epidermal change allows the distinction of tinea corporis from predominantly dermal annular lesions such as granuloma annulare and sarcoidosis.

Figure 12.24a and b Tinea capitis showing scaly lesions on the scalp. Scalp ringworm may lead to extensive alopecia, and in black children the likely fungus is *Trichophyton tonsurans*.

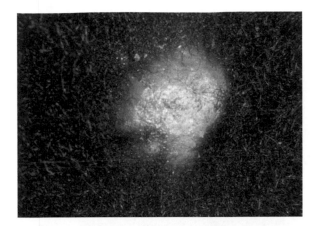

Figure 12.25 Kerion. This is an acute inflammatory response following infection of the hair shaft with *Trichophyton verrucosum*, usually seen in children after contact with cattle or domestic animals. The scalp is a common site but other hair-bearing sites may also be affected. A pustular folliculitis later becomes a boggy mass, accompanied by a scarring alopecia.

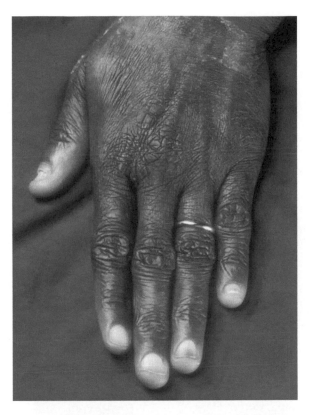

Figure 12.27 Tinea manuum, caused by *Trichophyton rubrum*, showing slight scaling and hyperpigmentation on the dorsum of the hand in a woman with deeply pigmented skin. Any species of dermatophyte may affect the skin of the hand. A large number of cases of tinea manuum are unilateral.

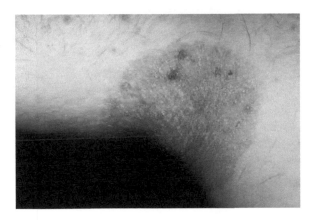

Figure 12.26 Tinea corporis, showing an area of tinea adjacent in the axillary region of an Indian patient, the lesion being hyperpigmented. Dermatophyte infections commonly affect the flexures (tinea cruris) when scaling may not be apparent.

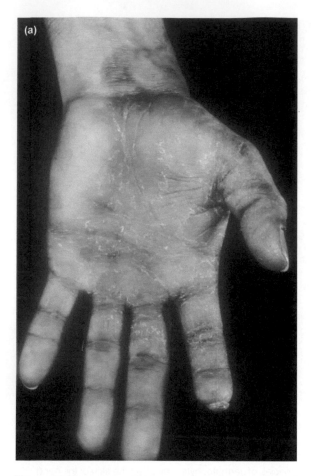
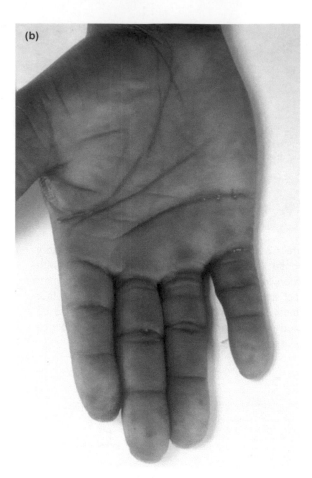

Figure 12.28a and b   Tinea manuum, showing diffuse hyperkeratosis on the palms and palmar surfaces of the fingers accompanied by hyperpigmentation and accentuation of the flexural creases (also seen as a normal variant in black skin, Chapter 1). 12.28b is an example of infection with the mould *Scytalidium hyalinum*, a variant of *Scytalidium dimidiatum* (previously known as *Hendersonula toruloidea*). These organisms are sensitive to cycloheximide and may be missed if this agent is used in routine culture media. These infections may coexist with a dermatophyte infection.

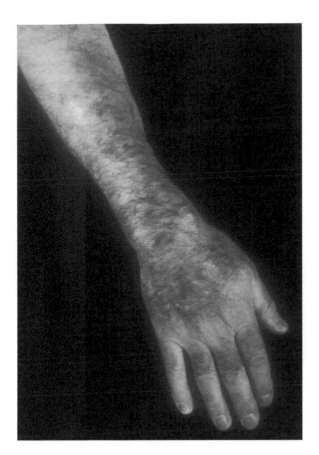

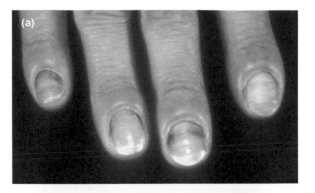

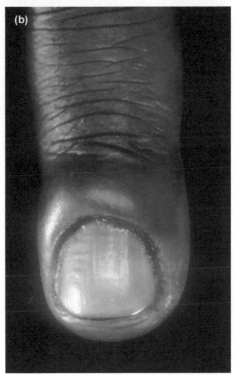

Figure 12.29 Tinea incognito, showing an extensive dermatophyte infection on the forearm and dorsum of the hand in a patient in whom host defence mechanisms had been impaired by the use of potent topical corticosteroids.

Figure 12.30a and b Candidal paronychia, showing inflamed boggy swellings of the nail-fold region in a white patient (12.30a). In a black patient (12.30b) the inflammation may not be discernable but gentle pressure on the swollen nail fold often causes the discharge of pus, from which a swab can be taken. Candidal paronychia occurs particularly in individuals whose hands are regularly immersed in water.

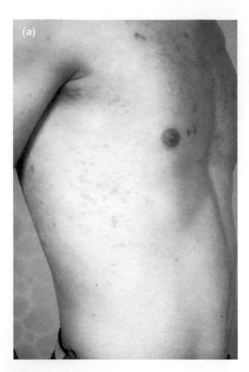 

Figure 12.31a and b   Pityriasis versicolor (tinea versicolor) on the trunk. In white skin, individual reddish slightly scaly lesions coalesce to form confluent areas (12.31a), hypopigmentation being the predominant feature in white people with a suntan (12.31b). Hypopigmented and hyperpigmented examples of pityriasis versicolor in black skin are shown in Chapter 1.

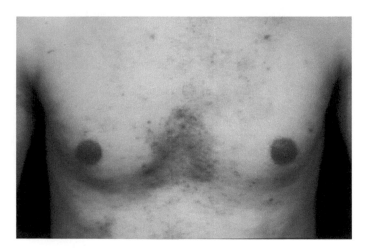

Figure 12.32   Pityrosporum folliculitis, showing red monomorphic perifollicular lesions on the chest of a white man. Hyperpigmented perifollicular lesions are shown in a black person in Chapter 3.

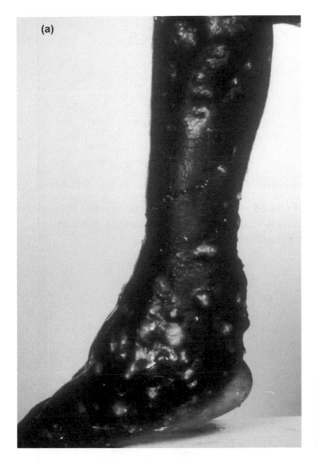

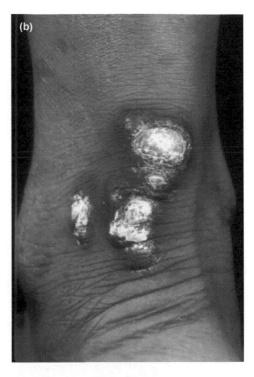

Figure 12.33a and b Chromoblastomycosis (chromomycosis), showing characteristic verrucous nodules on the lower leg (12.33a) and posterior ankle (12.33b) in a black person. Some of the lesions are reddish in colour and there is prominent hyperkeratosis.

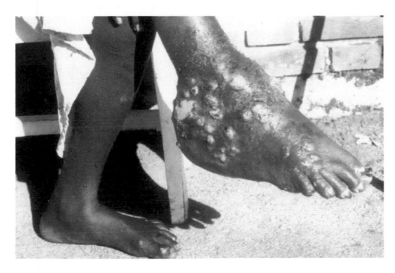

Figure 12.34 Mycetoma, affecting the foot of a patient of African origin. The infection is deep-seated and there are usually multiple granulomas, abscesses, and discharging sinuses.

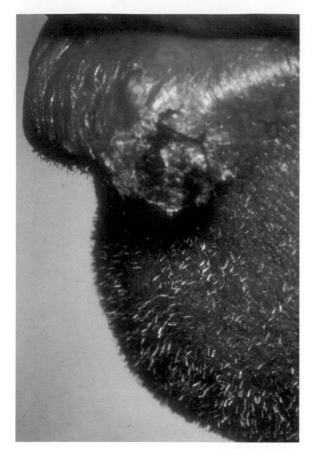

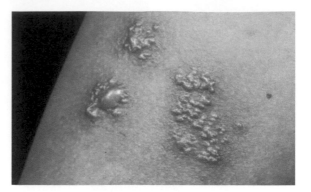

Figure 12.36   Herpes simplex, showing early grouped vesicular lesions with surrounding redness on the arm of a patient with black skin.

Figure 12.35   Coccidioidomycosis, showing a crusted plaque on the lower lip resulting from systemic infection of this primary airborne infection. Granulomatous papules, pustules, and nodules often appear on the face, scalp, or neck. Lesions may later form confluent plaques, necrotic ulcers, and verrucous granulomas.

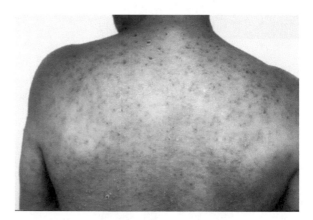

Figure 12.37   Chickenpox (varicella), showing excoriated papules and pustules on the upper back of a person with deeply pigmented skin.

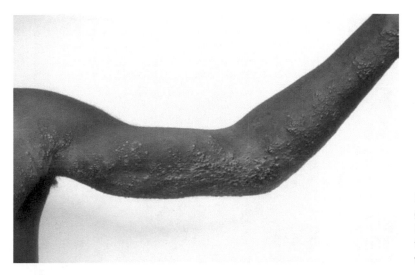

Figure 12.38 Herpes zoster (shingles), showing painful linear, vesicular lesions in a dermatomal distribution on the medial aspect of the arm of a man with black skin.

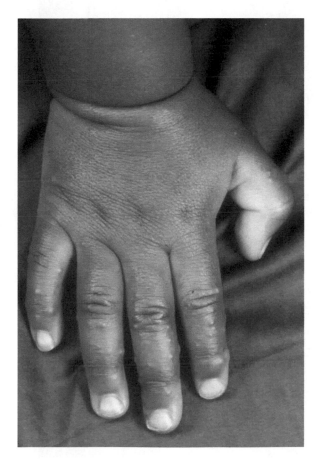

Figure 12.39 Hand-foot-and-mouth disease, showing blisters on the dorsum of the hand in a child with black skin.

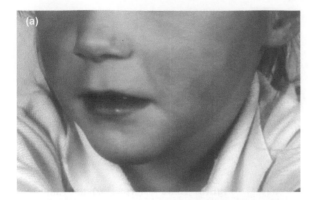

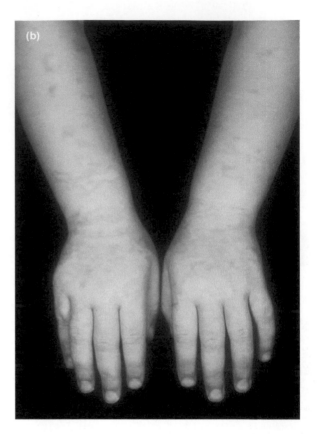

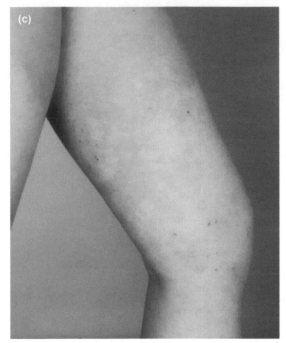

Figure 12.40a, b, and c   Erythema infectiosum (fifth disease), showing the characteristic 'slapped cheek' appearance on the face (12.40a) and the erythematous reticulate eruption on the limbs (12.40b and c).

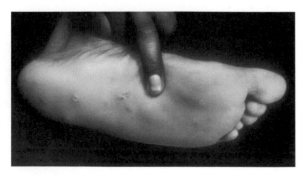

Figure 12.41   Viral warts (verrucae) on the plantar surface of the foot of a man with black skin. Note the lighter colour of the skin on the sole of the foot.

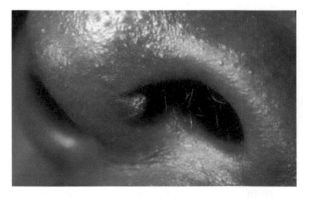

Figure 12.42   Viral wart, showing a filiform lesion in the left nostril region of a patient with deeply pigmented skin.

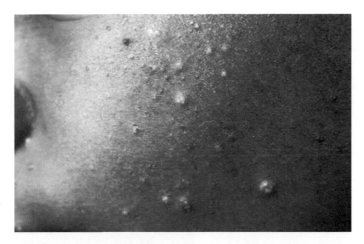

Figure 12.43 Molluscum contagiosum, showing several lesions on the left cheek of a person with pigmented skin. Some individual lesions have an umbilicated surface. In a healthy child molluscum contagiosum lesions eventually resolve spontaneously but sometimes large persistent lesions can cause great morbidity in immunocompromised patients (e.g. AIDS).

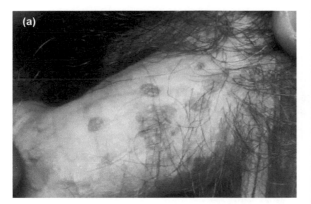

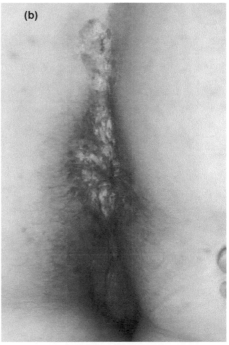

Figure 12.44a and b Bowenoid papulosis, showing numerous red papules and plaques on the penis (12.44a). The vulva and perianal region (12.44b) may also be affected by this multicentric disorder, caused by a human papillomavirus infection. This disorder should be distinguished from Bowen's disease and extensive surgery is not indicated in Bowenoid papulosis.

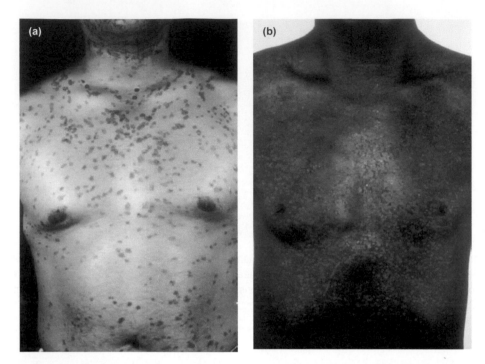

Figure 12.45a and b   Epidermodysplasia verruciformis, showing numerous reddish-brown plane warts on the anterior trunk (12.45a). 12.45b shows multiple coalescing orange-brown warts on the anterior trunk in a black patient.

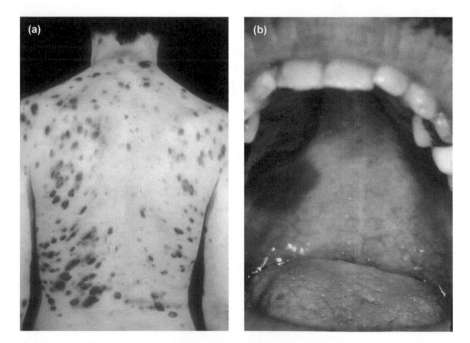

Figure 12.46a and b   Kaposi's sarcoma, showing numerous dark violaceous nodules on the back of a white man with AIDS (12.46a). The cutaneous lesions of Kaposi's sarcoma in this setting are often accompanied by haemorrhagic areas on the hard palate (12.46b). One should also examine the buccal mucosa and skin for opportunistic fungal infections.

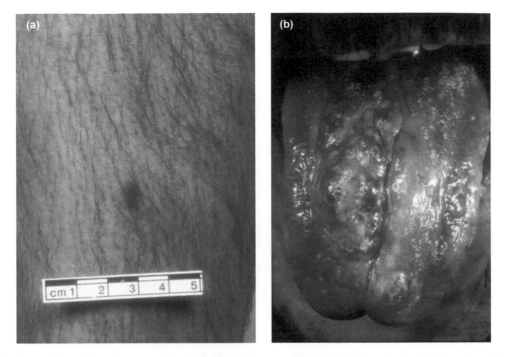

Figure 12.47a and b   Kaposi's sarcoma, showing a solitary nodule on the shin of a man with white skin (12.47a). 12.47b shows extensive vascular involvement of the tongue in a patient with AIDS.

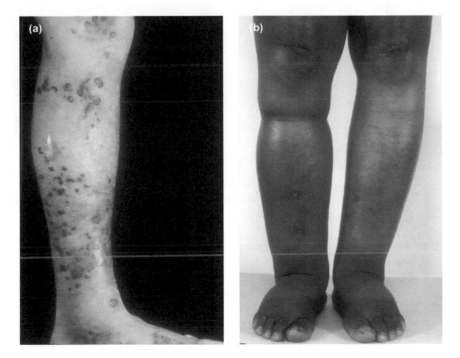

Figure 12.48a and b   Kaposi's sarcoma, the so-called classical type, as seen in patients without evidence of HIV-related disease. 12.48a shows purplish plaques on the lower leg and foot of an elderly white man. In black skin, there are hyperpigmented plaques, as seen on the lower legs and feet of an African man (12.48b).

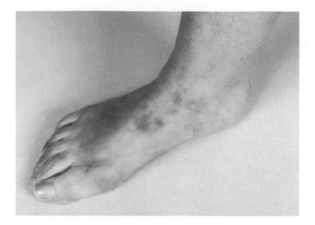

Figure 12.49 Cutaneous larva migrans (creeping eruption), showing itchy migrating serpiginous channels on the dorsum of the foot. The legs and buttocks are other common sites, reflecting contact of the skin with soil containing intestinal hookworm larvae.

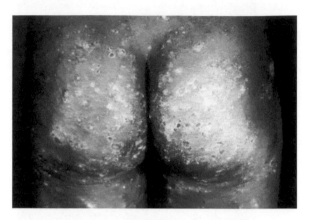

Figure 12.50 Onchocerciasis, showing excoriated hyperpigmented, lichenified, and hypopigmented lesions on the buttocks of a man from West Africa.

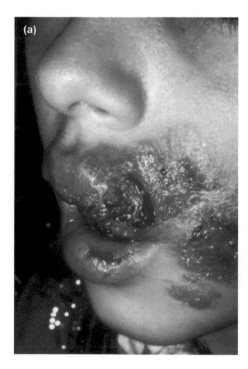

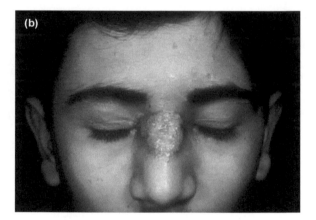

Figure 12.51a and b Leishmaniasis, showing ulcerated crusted cutaneous areas adjacent to the upper lip and extending onto the left cheek of a child (12.51a). 12.51b shows a healing plaque on the bridge of the nose in a young man of Indian origin.

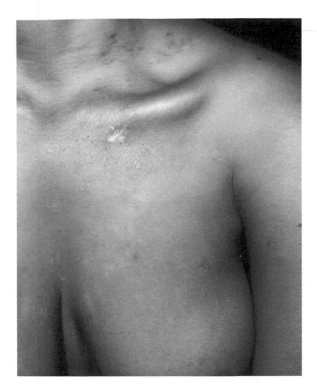

Figure 12.52 Schistosomiasis (bilharziasis), showing hyperpigmented papular lesions on the upper chest and neck of an African woman with ectopic cutaneous schistosomiasis. Other skin manifestations include schistosomal dermatitis, urticaria, and paragenital granulomas and fistulae.

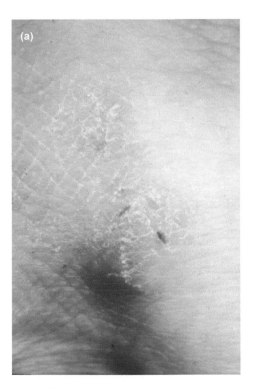

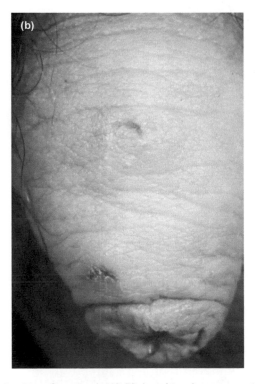

Figure 12.53a and b   Scabies, showing a linear burrow proximal to a finger web (12.53a) and two burrows on the penis (12.53b), both common sites.

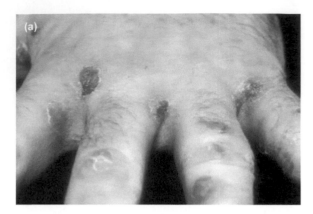
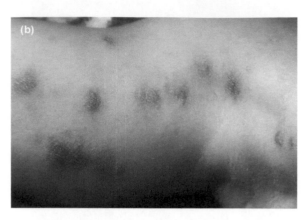

Figure 12.54a and b   Scabies, showing extensive secondary bacterial infection on the hand (12.54a). 12.54b shows reddish-brown lesions on the inner aspect of the upper arm and axilla in deeply pigmented skin; typical scabetic burrows were found at other sites on the body.

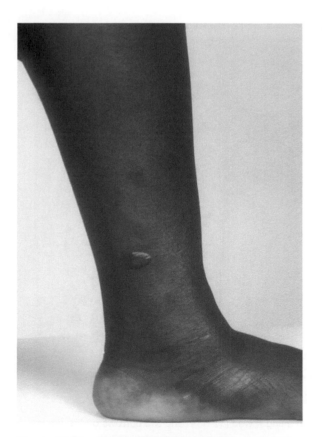

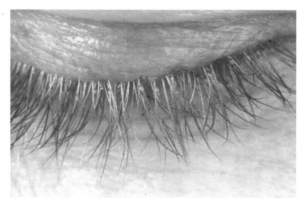

Figure 12.56   Pediculosis capitis is common in children with good personal hygiene, particularly in the school classroom environment. 12.56 shows an unusual finding of nits in the eyelashes of a person with head lice. In contrast, pediculosis corporis is associated with poor personal hygiene.

Figure 12.55   An itchy blistered insect bite on the lower leg of a West Indian woman.

Index

Pages with figures have suffix **f**, those
with tables have suffix **t**

acanthosis nigricans, 116
acarus hunt, 18
aciclovir, 77
acitretin, 21, 25
acne vulgaris, 2, 5, 16, 52, 57f
altered reactivity, 126–130
  drug reactions, 127–128
    Stevens-Johnson syndrome, 127
    toxic erythema, 127–128, 132f
    types of drug rash, 127
  other disorders of reactivity, 129–130
    aphthous ulcers, 129–130
    Behcet's disease, 130, 137f
    eosinophilic cellulitis (Wells' syndrome),
      129, 137f
    erythema annulare centrifugum
      (EAC), 129
    graft-versus-host-disease (GVHD),
      129–130, 136f
    Sweet's syndrome, 129, 136f
  photosensitivity, 128–130
    investigation of photosensitive rashes, 128
    therapeutic suggestions, 129
    second-line treatment, 129
    types of photodermatoses, 128
      actinic prurigo, 128, 135f
      actinic reticuloid, 128
      causative agents, 128
      chronic actinic dermatitis (CAD), 128
      polymorphic light eruption
        (PLE), 128
      porphyria cutanea tarda
        (PCT), 128–129
  polymorphic eruption of pregnancy
    (PUPP), 127
  pruritic urticarial papules, 127
  skin responds abnormally to stimuli, 126
  urticaria and angioedema, 126–127, 131f
    angiotensin-converting enzyme
      (ACE), 127
    effects of temperature, pressure and
      contact, 126

investigative tests, 127
reaction to food or drug, 126
therapeutic suggestions, 126
second-line treatment, 126
amyloidosis, 110, 116f, 117f
angiotensin-converting enzyme (ACE), 114
antibiotics, 55
antimalarials, 112, 134f
Archer, Clive, vii, 15, 19, 80
  personal view, 139
asteatotic eczema, 40f
azathioprine, 23, 77, 78, 80
azelaic acid, 52

basal cell carcinoma (BCC), 13, 15, 17
Behcet's disease, 130
benign melanocytic naevus, 14
benzoyl peroxide, 52
Berth-Jones, J., 26
BIE *see* bullous ichthyosiform erythroderma
Bilek, P., 19
*Black and White Skin Diseases:an Atlas and
  Text* (Archer and Robertson), vii
blistering disorders, 77–80
  bullous skin reactions, 77–78
    erythema multiforme, 77–78, 81f
      therapeutic suggestions, 77
      second-line treatment, 77–78
    oral ulceration, 82
    staphylococcal scalded skin syndrome
      (SSSS), 78
    Stevens-Johnson syndrome, 77–78
    toxic epidermal necrolysis
      (TEN), 77–78
  immunobullous diseases, 78–80
    bullous pemphigoid, 78
      specialist investigation of bullous
        diseases, 80
      therapeutic suggestions, 78
      second-line treatment, 78
    Hailey-Hailey disease, 85f
    immunofluorescence (IMF) table of
      diseases, 78, 79t
    pemphigoid gestationis, 84f
  mechanobullous diseases, 80

epidermolysis bullosa acquisita (EBA), 80
epidermolysis bullosa dystrophica,
  80, 86f
epidermolysis bullosa (EB), 80, 86f
pemphigus vulgaris, 78 82
Tzank smears, 79
Bolognia, J.L., 19, 26, 56, 68, 80, 90, 116,
  130, 142, 155, 168
Braun Falco, O., 19
Breathnach, S., 19, 26, 56, 68, 80, 90, 116,
  130, 142, 155, 168
Bristol Royal Infirmary (UBHT), vii
British Association of Dermatologists, vii
bulla defined, 3
bullous ichthyosiform erythroderma
  (BIE), 24–25
Burns, T., 19, 26, 56, 68, 80, 90, 116, 130,
  142, 155, 168

Campbell de Morgan spots, 88, 154
capsaicin, 24
CDLE *see* cutaneous discoid lupus
  erythematosus
Cerio, R., 19, 26, 56, 80, 105, 116, 130, 168
cheiropompholyx *see* endogenous hand and
  foot eczema
chest X-ray, 115
cicatricial pemphigoid, 83f
ciclosporin, 23, 78
clarithromycin, 162
clindamycin, 55
Clinical Investigation of Skin Disorders
  (Cerio and Archer), 26, 117, 168
clofazimine, 162
colchicine, 80
compression for venous ulcers, 103
contact dermatitis, 41f
corticosteroids
  induced atrophy of skin, 102f
  intralesional use, 87
  striae following long-term use, 102f
  topical use, 21, 23, 24, 25, 54, 55, 67
Coulson, I., 26
Cox, N., 19, 26, 56, 68, 80, 90, 116, 130,
  142, 157, 168

creatine kinease, 112
Crohn's disease, 104, 107f
Crotty, K., 19
crust defined, 3
cryotherapy, 87, 153–5
cutaneous discoid lupus erythematosus
    (CDLE), 55
cutaneous T-cell lymphomas
    (CTCL), 88–90
cyclophosphamide, 78

dapsone, 77, 80, 163
Darier's disease (keratosis follicularis),
    24, 25, 47f
dermal disorders, 87–90
  benign dermal disorders, 87–88
    dermatofibromas, 88
      leiomyomas, 88, 93f
      neurofibromatosis, 88, 93f
      tuberous sclerosis, 88, 93f, 94f
      xanthogranuloma, 88, 93f
    hypertrophic scar, 87–88, 92f
    keloids, 87–88, 91f, 92f
      acne keloidalis nuchae, 88
      therapeutic suggestions, 87
      second-line treatment, 87
    vascular lesions, 88
      ainhum, 88, 96f
      Anderson-Fabry disease, 88
      Campbell de Morgan spots, 88
      Jessner's benign lymphocytic infiltrate,
          88, 96f
      Osler-Rendu-Weber dfisease, 88
      port-wine stain, 88
      pyogenic granuloma, 88, 95f
      spider naevi, 88
  connective tissue diseases, 90
    Ehlers-Danlos syndrome, 90
    lichen sclerosus, 90, 100f
    morphoea, 90
    myxoedema, 90, 101f
    pseudo-xanthoma elasticum, 90
    therapeutic suggestions, 90
    second-line treatment, 90
  exogenous aetiology, 90
    therapeutic suggestions, 90
  glomus tumours, 88
  malignant dermal disorders, 88–90
    B-cell lymphoma, 89, 99f
    cutaneous T-cell lymphomas(CTCL),
        88–90, 97f
    follicular mucinosis, 88–89, 98f
    mycosis fungoides (MF) may be
        aggressive, 88, 97f, 98f
    investigation of MF, 89
    second-line treatment, 89
    poikiloderma, 89
    Sézary syndrome, 89, 99f
  dermatofibrosarcoma, 89

herpes virus, 90
  Kaposi's sarcoma (KS), 89–90, 100f
  Langerhans cell histiocytosis, 89
  monocytic leukaemia, 89
pretibial myxoedema, 90
dermal-epidermal cohesion see blistering
dermal-epidermal interface, 67–68
  chronic superficial scaly
      dermatitis, 67–68, 74f
  dermatitis herpetiformis, 83f
  lichen nitidus, 68, 73f
    therapeutic suggestions, 68
  lichen planus, 67–68, 69f, 70f, 71f, 72f
    therapeutic suggestions, 67
    second-line treatment, 67
  pityriasis lichenoides acuta, 75f
  pityriasis lichenoides chronica (PLC), 68, 76f
    therapeutic suggestions, 68
  pityriasis rosea, 68, 74f
    therapeutic suggestions, 68
dermatitis see also eczema/dermatitis
  chronic actinic, 44f
  contact, 41f, 42f, 43f
  lipstick, 42f
  nail varnish, 42f
  plant, 43f
  primary irritant, 40f
dermatological aspects of internal medicine,
    110–116
  acanthosis nigricans, 110
    clinical signs, 110
  amyloidosis, 110, 116f, 117f
    primary and myeloma-associated
        systemic amyloidosis, 111
      characteristics, 111
      therapeutic suggestions, 111
    primary localized cutaneous amyloidosis
        (PLCA), 110–111
  autoimmune and connective tissue disease,
      111
    Addison's disease, 111
    lupus erythematosus (LE), 111, 117f,
        118f, 119f
      discoid, systemic and subacute, 111
      hyperpigmentation and
          hypopigmentation, 111
      therapeutic suggestions, 111
      second-line treatment, 111
  dermatomyositis, 112, 120f
    electromyography (EMG), 112
    magnetic resonance imaging (MRI),
        112
    therapeutic suggestions, 112
    second-line treatment, 112
  granuloma annulare (GA), 114
    therapeutic suggestions, 114
    second-line treatment, 114
  mast cell disorders, 115
    therapeutic suggestions, 115

necrobiosis lipoidica, 115, 123f
  therapeutic suggestions, 115
  second-line treatment, 115
pruritus, 115
  may indicate systemic disorder, 115–116
sarcoidosis, 113–114, 121f, 122f
  common in black skin, 113
  granulomatous, 113
  investigation of sarcoidosis, 114
  therapeutic suggestions, 114
  second-line treatment, 114
scleroderma, 112
  characteristics, 112
  investigation of autoantibodies in
      connective tissue disease, 113
  lichen sclerosus et atrophicus (LSA),
      112, 121f
  morphoea, 112, 120f
  second-line treatment, 112
  xanthomatous disorders, 115, 124f, 125f
Dermatology: An Illustrated Colour Text, 26,
    56, 68, 80, 90, 142, 155, 168
dermatology defined, 1
diphencyprone, 55
discoid eczema, 39f
disseminated superficial actinic porokeratosis
    (DSAP), 49f
dithranol (anthralin), 22
Dunnil, M.G.S., 80

Eady, R.A.J., 80
eczema/dermatitis, 2, 21–24
Ehlers-Danlos syndrome, 90
electrodessication, 54
electromyography (EMG), 108
electron microscopy, 166
emollients, 25
endogenous hand and foot eczema
    (cheiropompholyx), 39f
epidermal appendages, 52–56
  acne, 52–53
    acne agminata, 58f
    acne keloidalis nuchae, 52–53, 88
    acne rosacea, 53, 58f
    perioral dermatitis, 58f
    pilosebaceous disorder, 52
    second-line treatment, 52, 53
    therapeutic suggestions, 52, 53
  cysts, 54
    epidermal and pilar, 54
    epidermoid cysts, 62f
    milia, 52, 54, 61f
    mucoid (myxoid) cyst, 64f
    steatocystoma multiplex, 63f
  Favre-Racouchot syndrome, 54, 60f
  Fox-Fordyce disease, 54, 60f
    apocrine gland disorder, 54
    second-line treatment, 54
    therapeutic suggestions, 54

hair problems, 54–56
  alopecia, 54–55, 64–65
    alopecia areata, 55, 64f, 65f
    alopecia neoplastica, 55, 66f
    cutaneous discoid lupus erythematosus
      (CDLE), 55
    folliculitis decalvans, 55, 66f
    second-line treatment, 55
    therapeutic suggestions, 55
    traction alopecia, 65f
    traumatic alopecia, 55
    trichotillomania, 55
  eruptive vellus hair cysts, 63f
  hirsutism, 54–56, 66f
    hyperprolactinaemia, 56
    hypertrichosis, 56
    pili torti, 56, 66f
    role of hormones, 56
    second-line treatment, 56
    therapeutic suggestions, 56
    polycystic ovarian syndrome
      (PCOS), 55
  hidradenitis suppurativa, 54, 59f
    scarring of the apocrine glands, 54
    second-line treatment, 54
    therapeutic suggestions, 54
  pseudofolliculitis barbae, 53–54, 59f
    caused by shaving, 53–54
    therapeutic suggestions, 54
    second-line treatment, 54
  rosacea and perioral dermatitis
    rhinophyma, 53
    therapeutic suggestions, 53
epidermal change, 20–51
  atopic dermatitis, 22, 36f
    characteristics and background, 22
    follicular pattern, 37f
    in infancy, 37f
    second-line treatment, 23
    secondary bacterial infection, 22
    therapeutic suggestions, 22
  contact dermatitis, 23
  eczema/dermatitis, 21–24
    characteristics, 21
    endogenous eczema, 23
    special investigation of eczema, 24
  eczema herpeticum, 37f
  inflammatory skin disease, 24
    actinic dermatitis, 24
    disseminate infundibulo-folliculitis, 24
    infantile acropustulosis, 24, 46f
    lichen simplex, 24
    lichen striatus, 45f
    nodular prurigo, 24, 44f
    therapeutic suggestions, 24
    second-line treatment, 24
  keratinization, 24–27
    acantholytic disease, 25
      therapeutic suggestions, 25

Darier's disease (keratosis follicularis),
    24, 25, 47f
Grover's disease, 25, 48f
Hailey-Hailey disease, 25, 85f
ichthyoses, 24
    bullous ichthyosiform erythroderma
      (BIE), 24–25
    collodion baby, 25
    harlequin fetus, 25
    ichthyosis vulgaris, 48f
    lamellar ichthyosis, 25
    link with X-chromosome, 24, 27f
    Netherton's syndrome, 25
    non-bullous ichthyosiform
      erythroderma (NBIE), 25
    persistent scaling, 24
    Refsum's syndrome, 25
  keratosis pilaris, 25–26, 48f
    acrokeratoelastoides, 26
    Flegel's disease (hyperkeratosis
      lenticularis perstans),
      25–26, 49f
    Kyrle's disease (hyperkeratosis
      follicularis), 25–26, 49f
    palmoplantar keratodermas,
      26, 50f
    porokeratosis, 26, 49f
    therapeutic suggestions, 25
    ulerythema ophryogenes, 25
  papulosquamous diseases, 20–21
    chnronic plaque psoriasis, 20–21
    genetic evidence, 20
    guttate psoriasis, 20–21
    pityriasis rubra pilaris (PRP), 21
      therapeutic suggestions
        and treatment, 21
    psoriasis, 20–21
      therapeutic suggestions
        and treatment, 21
    scaling papules and plaques, 20
    Sézary syndrome, 20–21
    use of skin biopsy, 20–21
  seborrhoeic dermatitis, 23
    common cause of dandruff, 23
    therapeutic suggestions, 23
    second-line treatment, 23
erosion defined, 3
erythema multiforme, 16
erythrasma, 18f
Ethiopia, vii
excoriation defined, 3
  second-line treatment, 3

facial Afro-Caribbean eruption
    (FACE), 154
Favre-Racouchot syndrome, 54
Flegel's disease (hyperkeratosis lenticularis
    perstans), 25–26, 49f
Fox-Fordyce disease, 54

Gawkrodger, J.L., 142, 155, 168
Glaser, D.A., 168
Griffiths, C., 19, 26, 56, 68, 80, 90, 116,
    130, 142. 155, 168
Grover's disease, 25, 48f

Hailey-Hailey disease, 25, 85f
Harper, J., 142
Heymannn, W.R., 26
hidrocystadenomas see syringomas
Hutchinson's melanotic freckle
    see lentigo maligna
hydrocortisone, 23

IMF see immunofluorescence
imiquimod, 153
immunofluorescence (IMF), 78, 80
infectious diseases and infestations,
    160–168
  bacterial diseases, 160–162
    acute bacterial infections, 161
      Bacillus anthracis, 161
      cellulitis, 160, 169f
      Corynebacterium, 161
      ecthyma, 160, 170f
      erysipelas, 160–161, 169f
      erythrasma, 161, 170f
      folliculitis, 161
      impetigo, 160–161, 169f
      necrotizing fasciitis, 161, 170f
      pseudofoliculitis, 161
      therapeutic suggestions, 160
      second-line treatment, 160
    cellulitis, 160
    chronic bacterial infections, 161–162
      fish tank granuloma, 162, 174f
      leprosy, 163, 174f, 175f, 176f
      Lyme disease (erythema chronicum
        migrans), 162, 172f
      papulonecrotic tuberculid,
        161–162, 173f
      pinta, 162
      syphilis, 161–162, 171f
      therapeutic suggestions, 162
      second-line treatment, 162
      Treponema pallidum, 161–162
      tuberculosis, 161, 162. 172f
      yaws, 162, 176f
    Staphylococcus aureus, 160, 161
    Streptococcus pyogenes, 160
  fungal diseases, 162–164
    deep (subcutaneous) fungal
      infections, 164
    chromoblastomycosis, 164, 183f
    mycetoma, 164, 183f
    sporotrichosis (from Sporothrix
      schenckii), 164
    therapeutic suggestions, 164
    second-line treatment, 164

investigation of bacterial and fungal diseases, 164
superficial fungal infections, 162–164, 178f, 180f, 181f
  athletes foot (tinea pedis), 162–163
  dermatophyte infections from *Trichophyton, Microsporum, Epidermophyton,* 162
  kerion, 163, 179f
  napkin candidiasis (from *Candida albicans),* 163
  pityriasis versicolor (from *Malassezia furfur),* 163
  scalp ringworm (tinea capitis), 163
  therapeutic suggestions, 163
  second-line treatment, 162–164
systemic fungal infections, 164
  aspergillosis (from *Aspergillus flavis),* 164
  coccidioidomycosis (from *Coccidioides immitis),* 164, 184f
infestations, 167–168
  insect bites, 167–168
  lice, 168
  scabies (from *Sarcoptes scabiei),* 167, 191f, 192f
  therapeutic suggestions, 167
  second-line treatment, 167
parasitic diseases, 166–167
  cutaneous larva migrans (creeping eruption), 166, 190f
  leishmaniasis, 9, 13f, 167, 190f
  onchocerciasis (from *Onchocerca volvulus),* 166–167
  schistososomiasis, 167, 191f
viral diseases, 164–166
  acquired immunodeficency syndrome (AIDS), 166
    Epstein-Barr virus, 166
    skin manifestations of AIDS, 166
  herpes virus (HHV8), 166
  human immunodeficiency virus (HIV), 164–166
  symptoms, 164–166
  investigation of viral diseases, 166
  Kaposi's sarcoma (KS), 166, 189f
  vesicular viral infections, 164–165
    herpes simplex virus (HSV), 164–165
      occurs in several clinical situations, 164–165
    herpes zoster (shingles), 165, 185f
    therapeutic suggestions, 164–165
    varicella (chickenpox), 165, 184f
  viral exanthems (measles), 165
  erythema infectiosum (fifth disease), 165, 186f
  viral warts, 165, 186f
    Bowenoid papulosis, 165
    epidermodysplasia verruciformis, 165, 188f

molluscum contagiosum, 165, 187f
papillomavirus (HPV), 165
types of warts, 165
Ingvar, C., 19
intralesional corticosteroids, 111
intravenous immune globulin, 112
irritant dermatitis, 40f
isotretinoin, 52, 54
itraconazole, 23

Johnson, E.M., 168
Jorizzo, J.L., 19, 26, 56, 68, 80, 90

Kaposi's sarcoma (KS), 89–90
ketoconazole, 23
knuckle pads, 51f
Koebner (isomorphic) phenomenon, 16, 113
Kyrle's disease (hyperkeratosis follicularis), 25–26, 49f

Langerhans cell histiocytosis, 89
Lebwohl, M.G., 26
Leeming, J.P., 168
lentigo maligna, 141
lesion defined, 3
lichen sclerosus et atrophicus (LSA), 108, 112
lichenification defined, 3
Lovell, C.R., 56, 116
LSA *see* lichen sclerosus et atrophicus
lupus miliaris faciei, 58f
lupus vulgaris, 16

macule defined, 3
magnetic resonance imaging (MRI), 112
malignant atrophic papulosis (Degos' disease), 105
McCarthy, W.H., 19
melanocytes, 138–142
  benign melanocytic naevi, 140, 146f
    naevus of Ota, 140, 149f
    naevus spilus, 140, 146f
    sebaceous naevi, 140, 148f
    Spitz naevus, 140, 147f
  decreased pigmentation, 138
    albinism, 138
    chemical leukoderma, 139
    hypomelanosis of Ito, 139, 145f
    idiopathic guttate hypomelanosis, 138–139, 143f
    post-inflammmatory hypopigmentation, 139
    therapeutic suggestions, 138
    second-line treatment, 138
    vitiligo, 138, 143f, 144f
  increased pigmentation, 139–140
    Albright's syndrome, 139
    Becker's naevus, 139, 144f

cafe au lait macules, 139, 145f
incontinentia pigmenti, 139
melasma, 139
post-inflammatory hyperpigmentation, 139
therapeutic suggestions, 139
second-line treatment, 139
malignant melanoma, 141–142, 152f
  superficial spreading melanoma, 141, 150f
  characteristics, 141
  lentigo maligna, 141, 151f
Menzies, S., 19
methotrexate, 21
miconazole, 23
Microsporum audouinii, 18
Microsporum canis, 18
minocycline, 104
minoxidil, 55
MRI *see* magnetic resonance imaging
Murphy, G.M., 26
mycophenolate mofetil, 78
mycosis fungoides (MF), 88

nail dystrophy, 65f
NBIE *see* non-bullous ichthyosiform erythroderma
nodule defined, 3
non-bullous ichthyosiform erythroderma (NBIE), 25
non-melanocytic tumours, 153–155
  benign skin tumours, 153–155
    benign dermal lesions, 154
      chondrodermatitis nodularis helicis (CNH), 154
      dermatofibromas, 154
      vascular lesions, 154
    benign epidermal lesions, 153–154
      actinic keratoses, 153, 156f
      dematosis paulosa nigra, 153, 156f
      facial Afro-Caribbean eruption (FACE), 154, 157f
      fibroepithelial polyps, 153
      milia, 153–154
      seborrhoeic keratosis, 153, 156f
    causes, 153–155
  low grade malignant skin tumours, 154
    Bowen's disease, 154
  malignant skin tumours, 155
    basal cell carcinoma (BCC), 155, 157f
    causes, 155
    Paget's disease, 155, 159f
    squamous cell carcinoma, 155, 158f
  therapeutic suggestions, 153
  second-line treatment, 153–154
nummular eczema *see* discoid eczema
Nurohy, G.M., 130

Oranje, A., 142

pachyonchia congenita, 50f
papule defined, 3
PCOS *see* polycystic ovarian syndrome
Penneys, N.S., 168
PG *see* pyoderma gangrenosum
pityriasis alba, 38f
pityriasis lichenoides chronica (PLC), 68
  therapeutic suggestions, 68
pityriasis rubra pilaris (PRP), 21, 26, 34f,
  35f, 36f
pityriasis versicolor, 18, 182f
pityrosporum folliculitis, 38f
plaque defined, 3
PLC *see* pityriasis lichenoides chronica
polycystic ovarian syndrome (PCOS), 55
porokeratosis, 49f
Prose, N., 143
PRP *see* pityriasis rubra pilaris
psoriasis, 2, 5, 8f, 20–21, 26f, 27f, 28f, 29f,
  30f, 31f, 32f, 33f
purpura defined, 3
pustule defined, 3
pyoderma gangrenosum (PG), 104

radioallergosorbent test (RAST), 22
Rapini, R.P., 19, 26, 56, 68, 80, 90, 116,
  130, 142, 155, 168
RAST *see* radioallergosorbent test
retinoids, 25
rifampicin, 55, 162
Robertson, Stuart, vii, 19
Rook's Textbook of Dermatology, 19, 26, 56,
  68, 80, 90, 116, 130, 142, 155, 168

Sarcoptes scabeii, 18
scabies *(Sarcoptes scabiei)*, 18
scale defined, 3
scar defined, 3
seborrhoeic dermatitis, 21, 38f
second-line treatment:
  acantholytic disease, 25
  acne, 52
  acne keloidalis nuchae, 53, 57f
  acute bacterial infections, 161
  atopic dermatitis, 22
  benign epidermal lesions, 153
  chronic bacterial infections, 162
  decreased pigmentation, 138
  folliculitis decalvans, 55
  hidradenitis suppurativa, 54
  inflammatory skin disease, 24
  leg ulcers, 103
  leprosy, 162
  lichen planus, 67
  photosensitivity, 129
  pityriasis rubra pilaris, 21
  pseudofolliculitis barbae, 54
  psoriasis, 21
  scabies, 167

seborrhoeic dermatitis, 23
  urticaria and angioedema, 127
Sézary syndrome, 20–21
skin biopsy, 15, 128
skin diseases and ethnic groups, 1–19
  clinical assessment, 10–12
  clinical investigations, 17–19
    dermatoscopy, 17
    malignant melanoma, 17
    seborrheic keratosis, 17
    Wood's light, 17, 18
    acarus hunt, 18
    examples of use, 18f
  common skin disorders, 2
  dermatological history, 12–14
    questions for the patient, 13
    'skin rash', 13
    sun exposure, 14
  dermatological problems in
      black skin, 4–9
    diagnostic difficulties, 4–5
      annular erythema, 4f
      annular sarcoidosis, 5, 6f
      granuloma annulare, 5, 6f
      pityriasis rosea, 5f
    pigmentary responses to disease or
        treatment, 5–7
      acne vulgaris, 5, 7f
      atopic dermatitis, 5, 6f, 10f
      depigmentation of vitiligo, 5–7
      exogenous (acquired) ochronosis, 6, 8f
      lichen planus, 5, 7f, 8f
      lupus erythematosus, 5, 7f
      pityriasis versicolor (tinea
          versicolor)), 6, 9f
      post-inflammatory hyperpigmentation
          (hypermelanosis), 5
      post-inflammatory hypopigmentation
          (hypomelanosis), 5
      psoriasis, 5, 8f
      vitiligo, 6, 9f
    prominent follicular and dermal
        inflammation, 7–9
      follicular eczema, 7, 10f
      infundibulo-folliculitis, 7, 10f, 48f
      keloids, 8, 11f
      leprosy, 8
  dermatological terminology, 3t
  diagrammatic view of the skin, 2f
  examining the patient, 15–16
    distribution, 16
      linear and grouped lesions, 16
      photographic evidence, 16
      table of skin disorders in
          body regions, 17t
    morphology, 15–16
      granulomatous changes, 15–16
      shape and colour of lesions, 15–16
    'window dermatology', 15

  general history, 14
    family history, 14
      allergies, 14
    past medical history, 14
    social history, 14–15
      atopic dermatitis, 15
  normal variants in black skin, 9
    asymptomatic pigmentation, 9, 11f
    cupping produces hyperpigmented
        lesions, 9, 12f
    Futcher (Voigt) line of
        demarcation, 9, 12f
    hyperpigmented macules on feet, 9, 12f
    leishmaniasis, 9, 13f, 190f
    leprosy, 9, 13f
    nail pigmentation, 9, 12f
    palmar pits (keratosis punctata), 9, 11f
  range of pigmented skin groups, 1–2
  skin pigmentation, 2–4
    melanin production, 2–4
    skin types with sun reactivity and
        pigmentary response, 4t
  table of skin diseases according to level of
      pathology, 3t
SSSS *see* staphylococcal scalded skin
    syndrome
St John's Institute of Dermatology, St
    Thomas' Hospital, London, vii
staphylococcal scalded skin
    syndrome (SSSS), 78
Staphylococcus aureus, 55
Stolz, W., 19
strawberry naevus, 94f, 95f
syringomas, 54, 61f

telangiectasia, 3
TEN *see* toxic epidermal necrolysis
tetracyclines, 53, 68
Textbook of Paediatric Dermatology
    (Harper), 142
thalidomide, 77
therapeutic suggestions:
  acantholytic disease, 25
  acne, 52
  acne keloidalis, 53, 57f
  acute bacterial infections, 161
  alopecia, 55
  amyloidosis, 111
  atopic dermatitis, 22
  benign dermal lesions, 154
  benign epidermal lesions, 153
  Bowen's disease, 154
  chronic bacterial infections, 162
  compression for venous ulcers, 103
  decreased pigmentation, 138
  epidermolysis bullosa, 80
  exposure to solar radiation, 111
  folliculitis decalvans, 55
  hidradenitis suppurativa, 54

immunobullous diseases, 78
inflammatory skin disease, 24
keratosis pilaris, 25
leg ulcers, 103
leprosy, 162
lichen nitidus, 68
lichen planus, 67
lupus erythematosus, 111
pemphigus vulgaris, 80
photosensitivity, 129
pityriasis lichenoides, 68
pityriasis rosea, 68
pityriasis rubra pilaris, 21
pseudofolliculitis barbae, 54
psoriasis, 21
scabies, 167
seborrhoeic dermatitis, 23
Sweet's syndrome, 129
urticaria and angioedema, 126
Tickman, M.J., 8
toxic epidermal necrolysis (TEN), 77–78
*Treatment of Skin Disease: Comprehensive
Therapeutic Strategies,* 26

Trichophyton schoenleinii, 18
trichotillomania, 55, 66f
Tzanck smear, 79, 166

ulcer defined, 3
ultraviolet B radiation (UV-B), 21, 23, 24, 127
urticaria, 2, 16

vasculature and subcutaneous
    disorders, 103–105
  skin ulceration, 103
    leg ulcers and pressure sores, 103, 106f
      therapeutic suggestions, 103
      second-line treatment, 103
      ultrasound studies, 103
    pyoderma gangrenosum (PG),
        104, 107f
      characteristics, 104
      therapeutic suggestions, 104
      second-line treatment, 104
  subcutaneous disorders, 105
    erythema nodosum, 105, 108f
    lipodystrophy, 105

    malignant atrophic papulosis (Degos'
        disease), 105
    panniculitis, 105, 108f
    Weber-Christian syndrome, 105
  vasculitis, 104–105, 107f
    arterial ischaemia, 106f
    chilblain, 105, 107f, 109f
    chronic venous insufficiency, 106f
    examples of lymphocytic vasculitis, 105
    inflammation of blood vessels, 104–105
    investigation, 104–105
      diagnosis, cause and systemic
          involvement, 104
      occurrence of palpable purpura, 105
      therapeutic suggestions, 105
      second-line treatment, 105
    Wegener's granulomatosis, 105
vesicle defined, 3
Vitamin D analogues, 21

Warnock, D.W., 168
wheal defined, 3
Wood's light, 17, 18

T - #0526 - 071024 - C208 - 254/190/10 - PB - 9780367386634 - Gloss Lamination